Psychosis in the Elderly

Psychosis in the Elderly

Edited by

Anne Hassett
Department of Psychiatry
University of Melbourne and
North West Aged Persons Mental Health Program
Sunshine Hospital
Victoria, Australia

David Ames
Department of Psychiatry
University of Melbourne and
St. George's Hospital
Victoria, Australia

Edmond Chiu
Department of Psychiatry
University of Melbourne and
St George's Hospital
Victoria, Australia

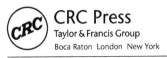

CRC Press
Taylor & Francis Group
Boca Raton London New York

CRC Press is an imprint of the
Taylor & Francis Group, an **informa** business

CRC Press
Taylor & Francis Group
6000 Broken Sound Parkway NW, Suite 300
Boca Raton, FL 33487-2742

First issued in paperback 2019

© 2005 by Taylor & Francis Group, LLC
CRC Press is an imprint of Taylor & Francis Group, an Informa business

No claim to original U.S. Government works

ISBN-13: 978-1-84184-394-0 (hbk)
ISBN-13: 978-0-367-39263-5 (pbk)

Although every effort has been made to ensure that drug doses and other information are presented accurately in this publication, the ultimate responsibility rests with the prescribing physician. Neither the publishers nor the authors can be held responsible for errors or for any consequences arising from the use of information contained herein. For detailed prescribing information or instructions on the use of any product or procedure discussed herein, please consult the prescribing information or instructional material issued by the manufacturer.

A CIP record for this book is available from the British Library.

Library of Congress Cataloging-in-Publication Data

Data available on application

Composition by J&L Composition, Filey, North Yorkshire, UK

Visit the Taylor & Francis Web site at
http://www.taylorandfrancis.com

and the CRC Press Web site at
http://www.crcpress.com

Contents

II. MANAGEMENT OF EARLY- AND LATE-ONSET SCHIZOPHRENIA

III. OTHER PSYCHOTIC DISORDERS IN THE ELDERLY

Contributors

Osvaldo P. Almeida
School of Psychiatry and Clinical
Neurosciences
University of Western Australia
Perth, Western Australia

David Ames
Department of Psychiatry
University of Melbourne and
St. George's Hospital, Victoria
Kew, Australia

Clive Ballard
Institute for Ageing and Health
Wolfson Research Centre
Newcastle General Hospital
Newcastle upon Tyne, UK

Ravi Bhat
Centre for Older Persons' Health
Goulburn Valley Area Mental
Health Service
Shepparton, Victoria
Australia

Richard Bonwick
Veterans' Psychiatry Unit
Heidelberg Repatriation Hospital
Melbourne, Victoria
Australia

Vincent Camus
Clinique Psychiatrique
Universitaire
Centre Hospitalier Régional
Universitaire
Tours, France

Amanda Carter
Normanby House
St George's Hospital
Kew, Victoria
Australia

David J. Castle
Mental Health Research Institute and
Department of Psychiatry
University of Melbourne
Parkville, Victoria
Australia

Edmond Chiu
Department of Psychiatry
University of Melbourne and
St George's Hospital
Kew, Victoria
Australia

Simon Douglas
Institute for Ageing and Health
Wolfson Research Centre
Newcastle General Hospital
Newcastle upon Tyne, UK

Lina Gibson
Normanby House
St George's Hospital
Kew, Victoria
Australia

Laszlo Gyulai
University of Pennsylvania Medical
Center and School of Medicine
Philadelphia, PA, USA

Anne Hassett
University of Melbourne and
North West Aged Persons Mental
Health Program
Sunshine Hospital
St Albans, Victoria
Australia

Dilip V. Jeste
Division of Geriatric Psychiatry
University of California
San Diego, California, USA

Rosemary Kelleher
Normanby House
St George's Hospital
Kew, Victoria
Australia

James Lindesay
Psychiatry for the Elderly
Leicester General Hospital
Leicester, UK

Christine McDougall
Normanby House
St George's Health Service
Kew, Victoria
Australia

Carlos Augusto de Mendonça-Lima
Instituto de Psiquiatria and
WHO Collaborative Center for
Research and Training in Mental
Health
Universidade Federal do Rio de
Janeiro
Rio de Janeiro, Brazil

Ramon Mocellin
Neuropsychiatry Unit
Royal Melbourne Hospital
Parkville and Melbourne Health
Aged Psychiatry Programme
Bundoora Extended Care Centre
Bundoora, Victoria
Australia

Trevor R. Norman
Department of Psychiatry
University of Melbourne
Austin and Repatriation Medical
Centre
Heidelberg, Victoria
Australia

James S. Olver
Department of Psychiatry
University of Melbourne
Austin and Repatriation Medical
Centre
Heidelberg, Victoria
Australia

Christos Pantelis
Melbourne Neuropsychiatry Centre
and Department of Psychiatry
University of Melbourne
Parkville, Victoria
Australia

Craig W. Ritchie
Department of Psychiatry and
Behavioural Sciences
Royal Free and University College
Medical School
London, UK

Heather Rota
Normanby House
St George's Hospital
Kew, Victoria
Australia

Martha Sajatovic
Case University School of Medicine
and University Hospitals of
Cleveland
Cleveland, OH, USA

Mary V. Seeman
250 College Street, Toronto
Ontaria, Canada

Dennis Velakoulis
Neuropsychiatry Unit
Royal Melbourne Hospital
Parkville, Victoria
Australia

Mark Walterfang
Neuropsychiatry Unit
Royal Melbourne Hospital
Parkville, Victoria
Australia

Catherine Waterhouse
Normanby House
St George's Hospital
Kew, Victoria
Australia

Greg Whelan
St Vincent's Hospital
Fitzroy, Victoria
Australia

Foreword

It is a great pleasure and an honor to have been asked to introduce this excellent book written partly by psychiatrists who have collaborated or studied with me in the past.

While delusions and hallucinations were central to psychiatry in much of the nineteenth and early twentieth centuries, exercising the attention of many of the great figures of the period, they came to be relatively neglected. Subsequently, attention focussed on disturbances of mood and memory and the search for causes and cures of these symptoms. More recent years have seen a revival in the study of the phenomenology of these disorders, the underlying structural and functional changes and their role in classification, diagnosis and treatment.

However, much new information has been spread about in relatively inaccessible publications. Insufficient attention has been paid to the links between late-onset psychoses, dementia, delirium and depression. The editors of this book skillfully bring together much of the important advances which have been reported on this subject extending from neuro-imaging to treatment, without ignoring important issues in epidemiology and classification.

An example of the way this has been handled is the chapter on the neurobiology of late-onset schizophrenia. The invention of computed tomography (CT) scanning by Hounsfield opened up the question of the relationship of structure and symptoms in psychiatry and especially in old age. The subsequent development of structural and functional magnetic resonance imaging (MRI) and positron emission tomography (PET) has allowed an even closer look at this issue in the psychoses of late life. Advances in molecular biology which have dominated much of medicine are applied with reference to late-onset persecutory states.

No aspect of this fascinating area of study has been neglected. The book should achieve a place as recommended reading for health workers in the field as well as those intrigued by problems which have beset psychiatry from its earliest days.

Raymond Levy
Emeritus Professor of Old Age Psychiatry
Institute of Psychiatry
King's College
London, UK

Acknowledgments

The editors would like to thank their personal assistants Roz Seath and Marilyn Kemp for their help with the preparation of this book.

James Lindesay wishes to thank Paul Bradley for his help with the preparation of Chapter 10.

Introduction

Clinicians caring for older persons have inevitably been confronted with patients presenting with a variety of clinical challenges relating to psychiatric symptoms in their patients. The usual concepts of schizophrenia whilst valid in the younger persons, do not always apply to their older patients. Paraphrenia sometimes seems a useful way of attending to a diagnostic dilemma but this too, frequently does not clarify.

Older persons have medical co-morbidities which impact upon or relate to the onset and trajectory of psychotic symptoms, adding additional challenges in the treatment of the whole person.

The Consensus Meeting at Leeds Castle which addressed the issue of schizophrenic illness in the older person gave us a valuable re-conceptualisation of this major psychotic condition and serves to bring to our awareness a total review in the understanding of what psychosis is in the older person.

In the years since the publication of the consensus report following the meeting, little has been published to bring together, in the same text, the whole range of psychotic presentations in the elderly. We hope this text will serve to clarify for the clinicians and researchers a range of psychotic presentations from schizophrenia-like psychosis through all other conditions in which psychotic symptoms are a part. It brings together both the biological, psychological and pharmacological aspects of this group of presentations, and adds to it the very important psychosocial, rehabilitation and community-based care of older persons with psychotic symptoms. Delirium, affective disorders, alcohol misuse and iatrogenic conditions are also included to address the relevant concerns of clinicians in the field.

As older persons with psychotic symptoms are much stigmatised in the community, this matter is also highlighted and addressed.

Recognising the field is sparse in the quantum of research and it is far less attractive to researchers when compared with the avalanche of work in dementia and depression, some future direction is drawn to interested researchers.

This text is offered to clinicians in the field and we hope to provide some assistance in their diagnostics and management of older persons with psychotic presentations. Above all, we hope to provide a better understanding of our older patients who suffer from and whose lives are blighted by these psychotic symptoms.

Anne Hassett
David Ames
Edmond Chiu

Melbourne, November 2004

chapter 1

Historical perspective

Mary V. Seeman and Dilip V. Jeste

Introduction

A small percentage of elderly individuals must, since time began, have felt spied upon by neighbors, cheated by families, invaded by intruders. According to epoch and place of birth, these expressions of what is now called delusional thinking were either dismissed as eccentricity, forgiven as frailty, or heeded as revelation. They almost certainly were not considered worthy of medical study until approximately the end of the nineteenth century. Since then, the classification of such symptoms in the elderly has varied, depending on how they were understood. Psychiatric classifications are never static but evolve over time, subject to changing concepts of health and disease. Vogues in diagnosis are always influenced by shifting theories of causation. Even the expression of symptoms, both in form (disjointed or coherent) and content (touched by God or hexed by evil spirits) varies over time periods. Social and historical forces inevitably put their stamp on symptoms and diagnoses (Markova and Berrios, 1995; Berrios, 1999; Zalewski, 1999).

Modern psychiatric nomenclature probably began in the late eighteenth century when the term 'neurosis' was first introduced. Neurosis referred to diseases of nerves and muscles and was initially attributed to a physical cause. The term 'psychosis', first used in the mid-nineteenth century, originally referred to a 'diseased mind' , a subgroup of the neuroses. By 1900, these two terms had taken on new meaning. Psychosis was now considered as a class apart, the outcome of brain pathology; neurosis was thought to originate in psychological conflict (Beer, 1996). As these changes were occurring, life expectancy began to rise and, over the course of the twentieth century, this continued dramatic increase in lifespan changed the social and cultural meaning of growing old. Until the end of the nineteenth century, the old were seen as preparing for death and it was chaplains, not doctors, who were called to care for them. By the late 1940s, old age had become a specific social and medical problem requiring professional help. When medicine and psychiatry finally turned their attention to diseases of the old, Foucault derided this new turn of events and called it the 'medicalization of old age', medicine arrogantly appropriating the terrain of sociology (Gockenjan, 1993; Hirshbein, 2001).

The definition of old age has changed over the years. One hundred years ago, those over 60 were considered elderly. This point of division was based on French and German statistics showing a decline in function beginning at that age (Kirk, 1992). Today, that line would be drawn later and very likely at a different age in different parts of the world (Stearns, 1981).

Late-life psychosis

Psychosis of old age at the beginning of the twentieth century thus meant a psychotic illness first emerging after age 60. The various categories of psychotic illness, quite apart from onset age, have undergone considerable change and discussion over the last 100 years (Jablensky, 1999; Eyler and Jeste, 2002). The distinction between the two major forms of psychosis, schizophrenia (dementia praecox) and bipolar disorder (manic-depressive insanity), proposed by Kraepelin in 1896, has been vigorously debated (Berrios and Hauser, 1988). The debate about nosology is most vigorous when applied to the elderly, among whom psychotic features are seen in conjunction with schizophrenia, affective illness, delusional disorder, delirium, and dementia. The onset of delusions and hallucinations in old age can arise de novo or can be associated with pre-existing mood disorder or newly acquired medical disorder or dementia. Whether the syndrome fits best under the rubric of schizophrenia or delusional disorder has been the subject of considerable controversy since 1955 (Roth, 1955; Karim and Burns, 2003).

The history of paranoia/paraphrenia

The ancient Greek word 'paranoia' (para noos) means 'beyond mind'. It was used in early times to describe madness. In the eighteenth century, it was a medical umbrella term for both mood disorders and dementia. The first systematic description of paranoid features with onset in later life was published under the title of *Involutional Paranoia* (Kleist, 1992). Kleist acknowledged that the clinical features of this disorder were very similar to those described by Kahlbaum in 1863 as paraphrenia.

An aside on the etymology of paraphrenia: When the heart was thought to be the seat of emotion, the term 'phrenum' (diaphragm) was used to describe the restraint placed on the heart. Paraphrenia thus meant 'beyond restraint' as in phrenetic. As the brain was ultimately understood to control emotion, 'phrenum' began to refer to the casing of the brain.

In the eighth edition of his 1896 textbook, Kraepelin subdivided paraphrenia into four forms:

(a)   paraphrenia Systematica: an insidious development of delusions of persecution and exaltation
(b)   paraphrenia Expansiva: exuberant ideas of grandiosity and mild excitement
(c)   paraphrenia Confabulaloria: falsifications of memories
(d)   paraphrenia Phantastica: extraordinary, incoherent and changeable delusional ideas.

The concept of paraphrenia has always been controversial. By 1921, German psychiatry considered paraphrenia a form of schizophrenia while psychiatrists in the UK considered it a form of delusional disorder. 'Late paraphrenia' was introduced in the mid-1950s as the term to be used when these conditions first began over age 60 (Roth, 1955). The term was still present in the ICD-9 (WHO, 1980), but is not included in current diagnostic classifications (Naguib, 1991; Berrios, 2003). Using ICD-10 (WHO, 1992) diagnostic criteria, about 60% of those previously diagnosed with paraphrenia meet criteria for schizophrenia, 30% for delusional disorder and 8% for schizoaffective disorder. Because there seem to be no significant differences between the patients in the ICD-10 schizophrenia and delusional disorder groups in terms of age at symptom onset, sex ratio, response to treatment, single status, the presence of insight or sensory impairment, the usefulness of such distinctions in ICD-10 and DSM-IV (American Psychiatric Association, 1994) when applied to the elderly population is questionable (Howard et al, 1994).

Risk factors for old age psychosis

Not only is there continuing debate about the nosological status of late-onset psychosis, but there is also controversy about the particular risk factors that are associated with this entity (Jeste et al, 1995, 1997). Early cognitive decline is frequently seen in these patients, but there is no clear relationship with a dementing process. Sensory impairment (Prager and Jeste, 1993), social isolation (Weeks, 1994), and a family history of schizophrenia (Almeida et al, 1992, 1995a) have all been associated with late-onset psychosis, but they appear to exert, at most, a nonspecific influence. Women exceed men in late-onset psychosis samples by 6–10-fold and this imbalance is not fully explained by the greater longevity of women (Castle and Murray, 1993; Almeida et al, 1995b; Lindamer et al, 1997). Although imaging studies have pointed to brain abnormalities, these changes appear subtle and generally similar to those found in patients with illness onset in earlier life (but late-onset cases show more signal hyperintensities than controls) (Corey-Bloom et al, 1995; Sachdev et al, 1999).

Symptoms

Late-onset paranoid disorders have two main symptom characteristics: a preoccupation with the transgression of personal space (partition delusions), and delusions of personal injury (robbery, jealousy, infestation). These phenomena are present in over 50% of 'late paraphrenias' compared with a rate of 20% in schizophrenia of young adult onset. Social isolation and cognitive deficits have been cited as contributory (Howard et al, 1992).

The controversy and the attempts to resolve the controversy

Since the early 1960s, discussions about the nature of late-onset psychoses have focused on two conflicting views:

(a) that they are the expression of schizophrenia in the elderly
(b) that they are genetically different from schizophrenia and arise from the complex interaction of various vulnerability factors associated with old age.

Besides the confusion between delusional disorders and schizophrenic disorders in old age, there is also the confusion between late-life paranoid disorders and Alzheimer's disease (AD), as both show some similar brain changes, although to different degrees (Förstl et al, 1994). Approximately 50% of patients with AD experience delusions or hallucinations within 3 years of clinical diagnosis (Jeste and Finkel, 2000; Paulsen et al, 2000). Psychosis is more likely to present during intermediate stages of dementia than in very early or very late stages. Another confusion arises between delusional disorders and affective disorders, first noted by Kraepelin, particularly between mania and 'paraphrenia confabulans'. Since Kraepelin, German psychiatry has focused on the similarities of symptoms and course of these two entities, much as it has focused on the similarities between schizophrenia and paranoid disorders of old age (Riecher-Rössler et al, 1995). French psychiatry, on the other hand, considers paraphrenia to be the end product of a prior psychotic disorder, such as mania (Sarfati et al, 1997). Adding to the complexity of sorting out nosological entities are the co-morbid physical illnesses, social isolation, sensory deficits, cognitive changes, effects of polypharmacy, and substance abuse often suffered by the elderly (Targum and Abbott, 1999).

To resolve controversies such as these, a two-day international meeting was held at Leeds Castle outside London in July 1998 to attempt a consensus on terms. The debates at the meeting plus a review of the literature achieved the following agreement: The term paraphrenia is best dropped. Nonorganic, nonaffective psychoses that have a first onset in later life can be divided epidemiologically into two categories: (a) late-onset schizophrenia (illness onset after 40 years of age but otherwise indistinguishable from schizophrenia starting at an earlier age) and, (b) very-late-onset schizophrenia-like psychosis (onset after 60 years). This latter group is generally associated with a somewhat different symptom profile and does not seem to have genetic risk factors for schizophrenia (Howard et al, 1997, 2000; Roth and Kay, 1998; Hafner et al, 2001; Palmer et al, 2001; Howard and Reeves, 2003).

Epidemiology

For the so-called 'functional' psychoses of late life, epidemiological information comes from two sources: studies of persons who have reached psychiatric services and surveys of elderly persons sampled from the general population. Except in terms of numbers affected, there is no notable divergence in the information obtained from clinical series and from population-based surveys. Late-life-onset psychotic symptoms are present in nearly 10% of patients over 65 attending a psychogeriatric clinic and are positively associated with increasing age. About three-quarters of patients are women, usually in their seventies. A study designed to identify prospectively patients suffering from very-late-onset schizophrenia-like psychosis (VLOSLP) recently enrolled 21 VLOSLP patients (15 women, 6 men; mean age, 78.1 years) and 21 age- and gender-matched elderly schizophrenia patients. The VLOSLP group was characterized by higher education, a higher rate of marriage, more pronounced cerebellar atrophy, and better response to treatment with risperidone (Barak et al, 2002).

Psychosocial issues

Despite speculations about the influence on symptoms of the failure to achieve resolution of developmental tasks (Hassett, 1997, 2003; Webster and Grossberg, 1998), the psychological aspects of both etiology and treatment of late-onset forms of psychosis have received relatively little attention (Aguera-Ortiz and Reneses-Prieto, 2003). Alcohol problems in old age that may contribute to psychotic symptoms have also not received adequate consideration (Johnson, 2000).

Conclusions

The onset of schizophrenia is typically during late adolescence or early adulthood; however, approximately a quarter to a fifth of patients manifest symptoms for the first time in middle or old age. Inconsistencies in nosology have resulted in diagnostic confusion in these cases. There are no clinical or laboratory tests that can reliably establish or rule out schizophrenia (in contrast to computed tomography (CT) or magnetic resonance imaging (MRI) for a large brain tumor). An international consensus conference involving researchers in the area of psychotic disorders in late life recently concluded that there was empirical support for the notion of two groups: late-onset (mostly middle-age-onset) schizophrenia and VLOSLP.

A number of investigations in different parts of the world have demonstrated that patients meeting strict clinical criteria for late-onset schizophrenia are similar to those with early-onset schizophrenia in symptoms, family history, pattern of neuropsychological impairment, nonspecific CT or MRI abnormalities, chronicity, and overall qualitative response to treatments such as antipsychotics. Furthermore, these patients do not meet criteria for mood disorders or dementia even when followed over a number of years. These strong similarities support a diagnosis of schizophrenia in the late-onset (mostly middle-age-onset) group. At the same time, there are several noteworthy differences between early- versus late-onset schizophrenia that suggest that the latter should be identified as a distinct subtype of schizophrenia – e.g. a higher prevalence of late-onset schizophrenia in women, its association with paranoid symptoms, less severe cognitive impairment, and improvement with lower doses of antipsychotics. Finally, a distinction between patients with middle-age-onset schizophrenia and geriatric-onset psychoses in terms of epidemiological, etiological, and symptom characteristics suggests that VLOSLP is a separate category. It differs from both early- and late- (i.e. middle-age-onset) schizophrenia in being associated with sensory impairment, social isolation, and visual hallucinations (Spitzer et al, 1978; Rabins et al, 1984), but not with formal thought disorder, affective blunting, or familial aggregation of schizophrenia. There is a need for continued research in further refining the proposed new nosologic schema.

References

Aguera-Ortiz L, Reneses-Prieto B, Practical psychological management of old age psychosis, *J Nutr Health Aging* (2003) 7:412–20.

Almeida OP, Howard R, Förstl H et al, Late paraphrenia: a review, *Int J Geriatr Psychiatry* (1992) 7:543–8.

Almeida OP, Howard RJ, Levy R et al, Psychotic states arising in late life (late paraphrenia): psychopathology and nosology, *Br J Psychiatry* (1995a) 165:205–14.

Almeida OP, Howard RJ, Levy R et al, Psychotic states arising in late life (late paraphrenia): the role of risk factors, *Br J Psychiatry* (1995b) 166:215–28.

American Psychiatric Association, *Diagnostic and Statistical Manual of Mental Disorders*, 4th edn (DSM–IV) (American Psychiatric Association: Washington, DC, 1994).

Barak Y, Aizenberg D, Mirecki I et al, Very late-onset schizophrenia-like psychosis: clinical and imaging characteristics in comparison with elderly patients with schizophrenia, *J Nerv Ment Dis* (2002) 190:733–6.

Beer MD, The dichotomies: psychosis/neurosis and functional/organic: a historical perspective, *Hist Psychiatry* (1996) 7:231–55.

Berrios GE, Classifications in psychiatry: a conceptual history, *Aust N Z J Psychiatry* (1999) 33:145–60.

Berrios GE, The insanities of the third age: a conceptual history of paraphrenia, *J Nutr Health Aging* (2003) 7:394–9.

Berrios GE, Hauser R, The early development of Kraeplin's ideas on classification: a conceptual history, *Psychol Med* (1988) 18:813–21.

Castle DJ, Murray RM, The epidemiology of late-onset schizophrenia, *Schizophr Bull* (1993) 19:691–700.

Corey-Bloom J, Jernigan T, Archibald S et al, Quantitative magnetic resonance imaging of the brain in late-life schizophrenia, *Am J Psychiatry* (1995) 152:447–9.

Eyler LT, Jeste DV, Late-life psychotic disorders: nosology and classification. In: Copeland J, Abou-Saeh M, Blazer D, eds, *Principles and Practice of Geriatric Psychiatry* (John Wiley and Sons: Chichester, 2002).

Förstl H, Dalgalarrondo P, Riecher-Rössler A et al, Organic factors and the clinical features of late paranoid psychosis: a comparison with Alzheimer's disease and normal aging, *Acta Psychiatr Scand* (1994) 89:335–40.

Gockenjan G, Medicine, old age and public interest in historical perpective: the German case, *Dynamis* (1993) 13:55–71.

Häfner H, Löffler W, Riecher-Rössler A et al, Schizophrenia and delusions in middle-aged and elderly patients: epidemiology and etiological hypothesis, *Nervenarzt* (2001) 72:347–57.

Hassett A, The case for a psychological perspective on late-onset psychosis, *Austr N Z Psychiatry* (1997) 31:68–75.

Hassett A, Psychosis and schizophrenic disorders in the elderly: an exploration of psychosocial factors which may influence emergence in late life, *J Nutr Health Aging* (2003) 7:401–8.

Hirshbein LD, Popular views of old age in America, 1900–1950, *J Amer Geriatr Soc* (2001) 49:1555–60.

Howard R, Reeves S, Psychosis and schizophrenia-like disorders in the elderly, *J Nutr Health Aging* (2003) 7:410–11.

Howard R, Almeida O, Levy R, Phenomenology, demography and diagnosis in late paraphrenia, *Psychol Med* (1994) 24:397–410.

Howard R, Castle D, O'Brien J et al, Permeable walls, floors, ceilings, and doors: partition delusions in late paraphrenia, *Int J Geriatr Psychiatry* (1992) 7:719–24.

Howard R, Graham C, Sham P et al, A controlled family study of late-onset non-affective psychosis (late paraphrenia), *Br J Psychiatry* (1997) **170**:511–14.

Howard R, Rabins PV, Seeman MV et al, Late-onset schizophrenia and very-late-onset schizophrenia-like psychois: an international consensus, *Am J Psychiatry* (2000) 157:172–8.

Jablensky A, The conflict of the nosologists: views on schizophrenia and manic-depressive illness in the early part of the 20th century, *Schizophr Res* (1999) 39:95–100.

Jeste DV, Finkel SI, Psychosis of Alzheimer's disease and related dementias: diagnostic criteria for a distinct syndrome, *Am J Geriatr Psychiatry* (2000) 8:29–34.

Jeste DV, Harris MJ, Krull A et al, Clinical and neuropsychological characteristics of patients with late-onset schizophrenia, *Am J Psychiatry* (1995) 152:722–30.

Jeste DV, Symonds LL, Harris MJ et al, Non-dementia non-praecox dementia praecox? Late-onset schizophrenia, *Am J Geriatr Psychiatry* (1997) 5:302–17.

Johnson I, Alcohol problems in old age: a review of recent epidemiological research, *Int J Geriatr Psychiatry* (2000) **15**:575–81.

Kahlbaum KL, *Die Gruppiening der psychischen Krankheiten und die Einteilung der Seelenströrungen* (Kafemann Verlag: Danzig, 1863).

Karim S, Burns A, The biology of psychosis in older people, *J Geriatr Psychiatry Neurol* (2003) 16:207–12.

Kirk H, Images of aging – over the last 100 years, *Dan Med Bull* (1992) 39:202–3.

Kleist K, Is involutional paranoia due to an organic-destructive brain process? Die involutionsparanoia. Allgenteine Zeitschriff für Psychiatrie (translated by Förstl H, Howard R, Almeida OP, et al.). In: Katona C, Levy R, eds, *Delusions and Hallucination in Old Age* (Gaskell: London, 1992) 165–6.

Kraepelin E, *Psychiatrie Ein Lehrbuch für sturdirende und Aerzte Fünfte, vollständig umgearbeitete Auflage* (Barth Verlag: Leipzig, 1896).

Lindamer LA, Lohr JB, Harris MJ et al, Gender, estrogen, and schizophrenia, *Psychopharmacol Bull* (1997) 33:221–8.

Markova IS, Berrios GE, Mental symptoms: are they similar phenomena? The problem of symptom heterogeneity, *Psychopathology* (1995) 28:147–57.

Naguib M, Paraphrenia revisited, *Br J Hosp Med* (1991) 46:371–5.

Palmer BW, McClure F, Jeste DV, Schizophrenia in late-life: findings challenge traditional concepts, *Harvard Rev Psychiatry* (2001) 9:51–8.

Paulsen JS, Salmon DP, Thal LJ et al, Incidence of and risk factors for hallucinations and delusions in patients with probable AD, *Neurology* (2000) 54:1965–71.

Prager S, Jeste DV, Sensory impairment in late-life schizophrenia, *Schizophr Bull* (1993) 19:755–72.

Rabins P, Pauker S, Thomas J, Can schizophrenia begin after age 44?, *Compr Psychiatry* (1984) 25:290–3.

Riecher-Rössler A, Rössler W, Forstl H et al, Late-onset schizophrenia and late paraphrenia, *Schizophr Bull* (1995) **21**:345–54.

Roth M, The natural history of mental disorder in old age, *Journal of Mental Science* (1955) **101**:281–301.

Roth M, Kay DWK, Late paraphrenia: a variant of schizophrenia manifest in late life or an organic clinical syndrome? A review of recent evidence, *Int J Geriatr Psychiatry* (1998) **13**:775–84.

Sachdev P, Brodaty H, Rose N et al, Schizophrenia with onset after age 50 years. 2: Neurological, neuropsychological and MRI investigation, *Br J Psychiatry* (1999) **175**:416–21.

Sarfati Y, Chauchot F, Galinowski A, Meta-process paraphrenia in manic-depressive disorder, *Encephale* (1997) **23**:459–62.

Spitzer RL, Endicott J, Robins E, *Research Diagnostic Criteria for a Selected Group of Functional Disorders* (New York State Psychiatric Institute: New York, 1978).

Stearns PN, The modernization of old age in France: approaches through history, *Int J Aging Hum Dev* (1981) **13**:297–315.

Targum SD, Abbott JL, Psychoses in the elderly: a spectrum of disorders, *J Clin Psychiatry* (1999) **60**(Suppl 8):4–10.

Webster J, Grossberg GT, Late-life onset of psychotic symptoms, *Am J Geriatr Psychiatry* (1998) **6**:196–202.

Weeks DJ, A review of loneliness concepts, with particular reference to old age, *Int J Geriatr Psychiatry* (1994) **9**:345–55.

World Health Organization, *International Classification of Diseases*, 9th revision (ICD-9) (World Health Organisation: Geneva, 1980).

World Health Organization, *The ICD-10 Classification of Mental and Behavioural Disorders: Clinical Descriptions and Diagnostic Guidelines* (World Health Organization: Geneva, 1992).

Zalewski Z, Importance of philosophy of science to the history of medical thinking, *Croat Med J* (1999) **40**:8–13.

chapter 2

Defining psychotic disorders in an aging population

Anne Hassett

Introduction

From a broad perspective, late-life psychotic symptoms can most obviously be classified as to whether they first developed in an individual's earlier years and have persisted, either continuously or in a relapsing manner, or whether they emerge for the first time in the context of a late-onset psychiatric or medical illness. In this chapter the separation of early- and late-onset psychotic symptoms will be the overall framework for examining these phenomena, as this approach is likely to have the greatest utility for the treating clinician in deciding on appropriate therapeutic interventions.

Early-onset psychotic symptoms

Individuals who 'graduate' into later life with psychotic symptoms most commonly have developed a schizophrenia-spectrum illness or severe affective illness (usually bipolar) in their early adult life or even younger. Psychotic symptoms in bipolar or unipolar affective illness are usually relapsing and develop predominantly in the context of periods of mood disturbance. The majority of these individuals have reasonable intermorbid functioning and have a relatively integrated social fabric to their lives. A minority, however, will experience significant disability because of poor response to treatment, rapid cycling and/or psychosocial deterioration. This will be discussed further in Chapters 12 and 13.

For those individuals who develop schizophrenia in early life the possible outcomes in later life are generally more heterogeneous. This has not always been the accepted view with regard to schizophrenia in late life, as Kraepelin conceptualized a core component of dementia praecox, being the inevitable and inexorable deterioration in an individual's personality and psychosocial functioning. However, long-term follow-up studies of patients diagnosed with schizophrenia have now disavowed clinicians and researchers of this notion and, perhaps, support the hypothesis that schizophrenia can no longer be conceptualized as a unitary diagnostic entity (McGlashan, 1988). In particular, five major long-term studies conducted in Europe and the United States followed more than 1000 patients diagnosed with schizophrenia for an average of 22–35 years. Recovery or at least significant improvement occurred in a half to two-thirds of cases (Gardos et al, 1982; McGlashan, 1984, 1988; Harding et al, 1987). Nevertheless, these studies confirmed that schizophrenia, if viewed as an overall illness entity, is chronic, disabling, and with an outcome that is generally worse than other major functional mental illnesses (Carpenter and Kirkpatrick, 1988). More recently, Cohen et al (2000) have highlighted that approximately only 1% of the literature on schizophrenia has focused on issues of aging, despite the fact that older persons with schizophrenia comprise the majority of those with serious and persistent mental illness. Further, these authors caution that we are moving towards an 'emerging crisis in mental health care' as the post-war baby boomers age and swell the numbers of older persons with chronic psychiatric illness, especially schizophrenia. Over the next 30 years this increase will be in the order of double the current population of aging individuals with a chronic psychotic illness. In particular, as a consequence of de-institutionalization, this generation of people with chronic mental illness has been treated predominantly in the community. Old age health and social service systems currently are ill-prepared for the increased demand on their resources that the 'baby-boomer' generation will create. If we are to effectively manage this looming crisis we need better to understand the likely consequences of long-standing psychosis for aging individuals, so as to develop management strategies that minimize the disability that is so often the outcome in chronic schizophrenia (Cohen et al, 2000).

So what happens to psychotic symptoms, the pathognomonic feature of schizophrenia, as an individual ages? Are they responsible for the deterioration in psychosocial functioning that befalls a significant percentage of individuals with this illness, or are aging-related factors, perhaps exacerbated by long-standing psychosis, more culpable in this regard? In order to provide a framework for understanding this area Cohen (1990) has divided outcome in late-life schizophrenia into three broad dimensions, one of which encompasses psychotic symptomatology, both positive and negative. Cohen (1990) emphasizes that the other two dimensions – cognitive/organic factors and social functioning – are closely interlinked with the outcome of psychotic symptoms in later life; so these three dimensions need to be examined as to their individual and inter-related contribution to outcome in later life.

With regard to positive symptoms, the elderly person with long-standing schizophrenia may have delusional beliefs, and/or perceptual disturbance (usually auditory hallucinations) and/or thought disorder. Ciompi (1980) observed that, although these psychotic features persisted into later life in chronic relapsing or unremitting schizophrenia, it was unusual for truly new positive symptoms to arise de novo at this life stage, i.e. the elderly person with 'graduate' schizophrenia usually continues to experience psychotic symptoms of similar form and content as when they were younger. If changes in positive symptoms do occur it is usually as a result of attenuation in the intensity and frequency of these phenomena. By way of explanation, Ciompi (1985) postulated that the aging process, perhaps in terms of developmental maturity, may exert a dampening effect on positive symptoms. This author also found that good premorbid adjustment, an acute onset, and a remitting rather than chronic course were factors associated with a reduction in positive symptoms in later life.

In contrast to positive psychotic symptoms, negative features such as avolition, affective blunting, and personality deterioration have been generally found to become more severe as the person with schizophrenia advances into old age (Cohen, 1990; Cohen et al, 2000). There is, however, controversy in this regard as some investigators contend that such symptoms also tend to remit in later life (Cohen et al, 2000). In particular, Cohen et al (2000) highlight that negative symptoms may be particularly difficult to identify in elderly schizophrenic patients because of the confounding effects of depression, demoralization, long-term antipsychotic therapy, and institutionalization. In a recent study of quality of life indicators in this group, Cohen et al (2003) found that negative symptoms, even more so than distressing positive symptoms, had a significant deleterious impact on the aging schizophrenic person in terms of their sense of 'subjective well-being'.

Closely linked with negative symptoms in chronic schizophrenia is the emergence of cognitive deficits and soft neurological signs. These may develop fairly early in the course of the illness, have a disabling influence on psychosocial functioning, and result in the aging person with schizophrenia experiencing a situation of 'double jeopardy' with respect to cognitive dysfunction (Cohen et al, 2000). That is, their cognitive resources are already compromised as they enter old age, which then leaves them with minimal reserve to cope with further age-associated cognitive decline or the co-morbid onset of a dementing syndrome. As a consequence, elderly patients with chronic schizophrenia frequently have some degree of cognitive impairment, and it is difficult for the treating clinician to determine to what extent this can be attributed to progressive negative symptomatology or a superimposed aging-related problem such as dementia. With the advent of cognitive-enhancing agents this diagnostic issue is rapidly becoming more critical than it ever has been in the past. For example, we now have ameliorative pharma-cotherapeutic options, such as the cholinesterase inhibitors, for our patients with a clinical diagnosis of Alzheimer's dementia. However, this is particularly difficult to detect in elderly patients with chronic schizophrenia, who are likely to have cognitive deficits associated with their chronic psychotic illness, but are also at risk of dementing at similar rates to the rest of the aging population.

With regard to the interaction of late-life chronic psychotic symptoms with social functioning, the clinician is presented with complex contradictory perspectives. On the one hand, elderly schizophrenic patients often have impoverished social networks, financial insecurity, and struggle with community-based living after years of institutionalization. Nevertheless, in later life there are likely to be fewer demands on their coping resources, and maturation and life experience may have helped them to achieve some 'co-existence' with their illness (Ciompi, 1985). As a consequence, they may experience less distress from their positive psychotic symptoms, and even may have achieved a degree of 'equilibrium' with their illness and disability (Cohen, 1990). However, because of the 'clinician's bias' predominantly we see those patients who do not cope very well with their illness, as they are most in need of ongoing monitoring and support. However, there are many older persons with schizophrenia who develop adaptive coping strategies that enable them to manage their illness and achieve some stability within their social milieu. Yet, there has been very little attention given to better understanding these coping styles. Cohen (1990) has emphasized the need for systematic study in this area, so as to enhance our understanding of adaptive psychosocial strategies associated with more favorable symptomatic and functional outcomes for the aging person with schizophrenia. On the other hand, it has been well established that worsening negative symptoms are significantly associated with social and functional decline in older schizophrenic patients. In particular, older males with chronic schizophrenia appear to be most at risk in this regard, and more likely to require long-term institutionalization at an earlier stage in their illness progression (Harvey et al, 2003).

Late-onset psychotic symptoms

In contrast to the elderly person with a well-established diagnosis of early-onset schizophrenia, the aging individual who becomes psychotic for the first time in later life frequently poses a diagnostic and management dilemma for the clinician. First, these phenomena occur across a broad spectrum of late-life syndromes and often are co-morbid with other psychiatric or physical pathology (Table 2.1). This prominence of psychotic symptoms across late-life psychiatric syndromes suggests that the aging process itself may be a risk factor for developing these phenomena (Van Os et al, 1995). Second, if cognitive deficits are present, the elderly person may not be able accurately to report the time-frame in which the psychotic symptoms emerged. This frequently is an issue in deciding if an elderly person is presenting with primarily a 'functional' disorder, such as schizophrenia, or primarily a dementing disorder with secondary psychotic symptoms. Collateral history is particularly important in these situations, but may not be available if the person is living alone and socially isolated.

Table 2.1 Psychotic symptoms across life stages

	Young	Middle age	Old age
Schizophrenia	+	+	+
Affective disorders	+	+	+ +
Alcohol misuse	+	+ +	+
Illicit substance use	+ +	+	
Delusional disorder		+	+
Specific organic		+	+ +
Delirium			+ +
Dementia			+ +

Third, as in psychosis arising at any stage of the lifespan, specific etiological mechanisms for the genesis of these complex phenomena have yet to be identified (Häfner et al, 1998). Thus, we have to rely on diagnoses made from syndromal constellations of symptoms and behavior that lack construct validity. This is particularly true for schizophrenia-spectrum illness of late-onset, in contrast to a number of dementia syndromes which, at least, can be identified histopathologically at post mortem (Paskavitz et al, 1995; Arnold et al, 1998; Falke et al, 2000). However, a post-mortem diagnosis is not helpful to clinicians who have to make diagnostic and management decisions without this confirmatory evidence. For example, it is now recognized that some cognitive impairment is present in many elderly patients presenting with late-onset schizophrenia-like illness (Almeida et al, 1995a, 1995b; Corey-Bloom et al, 1995). In undertaking studies of this area a decision then has to be made as to the diagnostic separation between a so-called 'functional' disorder, such as late-onset schizophrenia, from an 'organic' disorder, such as dementia (Mulsant et al, 1993; Yassa and Suranyi-Cadotte, 1993; Almeida et al, 1995b). The Mini-mental State Examination (MMSE) (Folstein et al, 1975) is the most widely used assessment instrument for identification of cognitive impairment in elderly subjects who are likely to be dementing. Of note, several studies of late-onset psychosis (Naguib and Levy, 1987; Almeida et al, 1995a, 1995b; Jeste et al, 1995; Sachdev et al, 1999) also have undertaken more extensive cognitive testing once subjects had been recruited.

The clinical and research utility of the MMSE lies in its relatively reliable discrimination of 'organic' disorders, such as dementia and delirium, from 'functional' psychiatric disorders (Field et al, 1995). Thus, elderly psychotic subjects with MMSE scores greater than 23/24 are generally accepted into studies of late-onset schizophrenia, while subjects with MMSE scores below this established threshold are recruited for studies examining psychotic symptoms as part of dementing processes (Förstl et al, 1994). This categorical approach, i.e. taking an MMSE score of 23/24 as a 'point of rarity' in order to separate psychotic symptoms that are associated with dementing processes from those symptoms that arise de novo in old age, has been necessary to identify 'caseness' in studies of elderly psychotic subjects. In reality, there appears to be no such 'point of rarity', as cognitive deficits of varying severity have been identified in elderly individuals who present with psychotic symptoms, even when dementia is not the primary diagnosis (Almeida et al, 1995a, 1995b).

As psychotic symptoms associated with overt dementing processes are examined in Chapter 14, the following discussion will focus on elderly patients who present with the florid psychotic symptomatology typical of late-onset schizophrenia-spectrum illness. The paradigmatic presentation for the clinician is a socially isolated elderly female who may have some hearing impairment, and elaborates systematized delusional ideas involving some threat to her home (Herbert and Jacobson, 1967; Pearlson et al, 1989; Howard et al, 1994; Hassett, 2003). It was Roth (1955) who first noted that the persecutory themes of these patients typically involved being under hostile scrutiny by neighbors or others, or threats to remove the elderly person from their home. Herbert and Jacobson (1967) similarly found that home-related safety and security issues were the predominant delusional preoccupation in a study sample of 47 elderly late-onset psychotic females. Many of these subjects were described as having 'partition delusions', which the authors defined as 'the belief that somebody or something is operating in the ceiling above, the floor below, or beyond the wall separating an adjacent room and is interfering with the patient's life and circumstances' (p. 465). Other authors (Pearlson et al, 1989; Howard et al, 1992; Hassett, 2003) similarly have found this type of psychotic phenomenon to be relatively common in late-onset schizophrenia, with rates between 15% and 90% of study samples. Rowan (1984) gave the name 'phantom boarders' to the uninvited guests that these elderly psychotic women often believed were living in their homes.

Although delusions have been the most commonly described phenomena in late-onset psychotic states, hallucinations also have been frequently noted (Berrios, 1992). Several studies (Leuchter and Spar, 1985; Pearlson et al, 1989; Howard et al, 1994) have reported the multimodal nature of hallucinations in late-onset psychotic states, particularly the involvement of visual and olfactory modalities, as well as auditory hallucinations. Some authors (Kay and Roth, 1961; Post, 1966; Herbert and Jacobson, 1967) have queried whether this finding may be associated with aging-related organic deterioration in these sensory modalities. Examining this issue, Howard et al (1994) noted that, while visual impairment was significantly associated with visual hallucinations, hearing impairment was not necessarily associated with auditory hallucinations. This is consistent with early-onset schizophrenia, in which auditory hallucinations are the most common type of perceptual disturbance and, usually, are not accompanied by hearing impairment (Andreasen, 1990). Howard et al (1994) postulated that perhaps, at least for visual hallucinations, specific sensory organ pathology may have an important role in the genesis of psychotic symptoms. As hallucinatory phenomena are also common in early-onset schizophrenia (Andreasen, 1990), it would seem that prevalence rates of these phenomena are unlikely to be a distinguishing feature between late- and early-onset disorders. On the other hand, the sensory modalities involved appear to be more varied when onset occurs in later life.

Unlike delusional and hallucinatory experiences, which occur in both early- and late-onset schizophrenia-spectrum disorders, most studies have found that thought disorder occurs far less frequently in the latter. Pearlson et al (1989) found that only 6% of 54 patients with DSM-III (American Psychiatric Association, 1980) schizophrenia developing after the age of 45 had thought disorder, in contrast to 55% of 22 older patients with early-onset schizophrenia, and 52% of 54 younger patients with schizophrenia. Other studies (Hassett, 2003; Howard et al, 1994; Almeida et al, 1995c) have also found the prevalence of thought disorder in late-onset psychosis to be notably infrequent. In studies of earlier-onset schizophrenia (Liddle et al, 1990), the presence of thought disorder has been postulated to represent a separate 'subtype' to that characterized by delusions and hallucinations. This construct of psychotic symptoms suggests that there may be less phenomenological diversity in late-presenting schizophrenia-like illness (Table 2.2).

From another perspective, Jeste et al (1988) used the positive–negative dichotomization of 'schizophrenic' symptoms to compare patients with late- and early-onset psychotic phenomena. These authors found that the mean

Table 2.2 Clinical presentation of schizophrenia in late life

Early-onset	Late-onset
Delusions	Delusions
• systematized	• systematized
• non-systematized	• 'partition'
	• phantom boarders
Hallucinations	Hallucinations
• usually auditory	• multimodal
Thought disorder	Thought disorder
• common	• uncommon
Negative symptoms	Negative symptoms
• common	• uncommon

total score on the Scale for Assessment of Positive Symptoms (SAPS) (Andreasen and Olsen, 1982) for 10 late-onset patients was similar to that of 15 younger patients (and especially so for the subscales for delusions and hallucinations). In contrast, the younger and older patients did differ noticeably with respect to negative symptoms. The younger patients scored almost twice as high on the total score of the Scale for Assessment of Negative Symptoms (SANS) (Andreasen and Olsen, 1982), and all the scores on the subscales (affective blunting, alogia, avolition, anhedonia, and attention) were higher in the younger group. In a later study, comparing 25 patients over 45 years of age with DSM-IIIR (American Psychiatric Association, 1987) schizophrenia, 39 patients with the same diagnosis, and 35 normal controls, Jeste et al (1995) confirmed their earlier findings. The late- and early-onset groups were similar to each other on the SAPS total score and subscales, but differed significantly on the SANS total score. This finding was almost entirely accounted for by the much lower rating of the late-onset group on the subscales for affective blunting and avolition/apathy.

In conclusion, studies investigating psychosis emerging at different stages of the lifespan have demonstrated that, while delusions and hallucinations can emerge for the first time at any age, other features characteristic of schizophrenia (thought disorder, affective blunting, avolitional disturbance) appear to become less frequent with increasing age. Persecutory themes, particularly relating to the person's abode ('partition delusions'), are a prominent feature when psychotic symptoms first present in late life (Howard et al, 1992). The development of this type of delusional phenomenon does not appear to be entirely age-related, as elderly patients with long-standing schizophrenia do not have these preoccupations to the same extent (Pearlson et al, 1989). Further, hallucinations across a range of modalities appear to be more common in late-presenting psychosis (Pearlson et al, 1989), although studies in this area are still few in number. These findings raise questions about possible etiological differences when schizophrenia-like illness presents in later life. An alternative perspective is that aging-related factors may exert a pathoplastic effect, so that the same illness presents as phenomenologically different at different life stages (Tsuang et al, 1990; McGorry, 1991).

Although research examining psychotic symptoms as they present in later life is a burgeoning area, the findings to date, as discussed in this chapter, have created more questions than have been answered. That there appears to be a range of outcomes for both early- and late-onset schizophrenia-like illness suggests that that there may be heterogeneous etiological processes operating, both aging- and nonaging-related. On the other hand, the common co-morbidity of cognitive impairment with psychotic symptoms also suggests some overlap in the pathophysiological 'pathways' of these phenomena as they become clinically expressed (Förstl et al, 1994). Further, the role of psychosocial factors (social isolation, premorbid personality, rehabilitation strategies) in the genesis and outcome of psychotic symptoms in later life has received minimal research attention (Henderson and Kay, 1997). As the number of older people with schizophrenia-like illness, both early- and late-onset, increases dramatically over the ensuing decades, clinicians working with these elderly individuals are going to be significantly challenged by their management needs. As Cohen et al (2000) emphasize in their review of schizophrenia and older adults, policy-makers must begin to reorder research and service priorities to anticipate this growth.

References

Almeida P, Howard R, Levy R et al, Cognitive features of psychotic states arising in late life (late paraphrenia), *Psychol Med* (1995a) 25:685–97.

Almeida P, Howard R, Levy R et al, Clinical and cognitive diversity of psychotic states arising in late life (late paraphrenia), *Psychol Med* (1995b) 25:699–714.

Almeida P, Howard R, Levy R et al, Psychotic states arising in late life (late paraphrenia): psychopathology and nosology, *Br J Psychiatry* (1995c) 166:205–14.

American Psychiatric Association, *Diagnostic and Statistical Manual of Mental Disorders*, 3rd edn (DSM-III) (American Psychiatric Association: Washington, DC, 1980).

American Psychiatric Association, *Diagnostic and Statistical Manual of Mental Disorders*, 3rd edn (revised) (DSM-III) (American Psychiatric Association: Washington, DC, 1987).

Andreasen N. Schizophrenia: positive and negative symptoms and syndromes, *Mod Probl Pharmacopsychiatry* (1990) 24:1–42.

Andreasen N, Olsen S, Negative v positive schizophrenia: definition and validation, *Arch Gen Psychiatry* (1982) 39:789–94.

Arnold SE, Trojanowski JQ, Gur RE et al, Absence of neurodegeneration and neural injury in the cerebral cortex in a sample of elderly patients with schizophrenia, *Arch Gen Psychiatry* (1998) 55:225–32.

Berrios G, Psychotic symptoms in the elderly: concepts and models. In: Katona C, Levy R, eds, *Delusions and Hallucinations in Old Age* (Royal College of Psychiatrists: London, 1992) 3–14.

Carpenter W, Kirkpatrick B, The heterogeneity of the long-term course of schizophrenia, *Schizophr Bull* (1988) 14:645–52.

Ciompi L, Catamnestic long-term study on the course of life and aging of schizophrenics, *Schizophr Bull* (1980) 6:606–17.

Ciompi L, Aging and schizophrenic psychosis, *Acta Psychiatr Scand* (1985) 319:93–105.

Cohen C, Outcome of schizophrenia into later life: an overview, *Gerontologist* (1990) 30:790–7.

Cohen C, Cohen G, Blank K et al, Schizophrenia and older adults, an overview: directions for research and policy, *Am J Geriatr Psychiatry* (2000) 8:19–28.

Cohen C, Ramirex P, Kehn M et al, Assessing quality of life in older persons with schizophrenia, *Am J Geriatr Psychiatry* (2003) 11:658–66.

Corey-Bloom J, Jernigan T, Archibald S et al, Quantitative magnetic resonance imaging of the brain in late-life schizophrenia, *Am J Psychiatry* (1995) 152:447–9.

Falke E, Han LY, Arnold SE, Absence of neurodegeneration in the thalamus and caudate of elderly patients with schizophrenia, *Psychiatry Res* (2000) 93:103–10.

Field S, Jackson H, Hassett A et al, The ability of the Mini-mental State Examination to discriminate diagnostic entities in a psychogeriatric population, *Int J Geriatr Psychiatry* (1995) 10:47–55.

Folstein M, Folstein S, McHugh P, 'Mini-mental State': a practical method of grading the cognitive state of patients for the clinician, *J Psychiatr Res* (1975) 12:189–98.

Förstl H, Burns A, Levy R et al, Neuropathological correlates of psychotic phenomena in confirmed Alzheimer's Disease, *Br J Psychiatry* (1994) 165:53–9.

Gardos G, Cole J, LaBrie R, A twelve-year follow-up study of chronic schizophrenics, *Hosp Community Psychiatry* (1982) 33:983–4.

Häfner H, Hambrecht M, Löffler W et al, Is schizophrenia a disorder of all ages? A comparison of first episodes and early course across the life cycle, *Psychol Med* (1998) 25:351–66.

Harding CM, Brooks GW, Ashikaga T et al, The Vermont longitudinal study of persons with severe mental illness: II. Long-term outcome of subjects who retrospectively met DSM-III criteria for schizophrenia, *Am J Psychiatry* (1987) 144:727–35.

Harvey PD, Bertisch H, Friedman J et al, The course of functional decline in geriatric patients with schizophrenia: cognitive-functional and clinical symptoms as determinants of change, *Am J Geriatr Psychiatry* (2003) 11:610–19.

Hassett A, Psychosis and schizophrenic disorders in the elderly: an exploration of psychosocial factors which may influence emergence in late life, *J Nutr Health Aging* (2003) 6:401–8.

Henderson A, Kay D, The epidemiology of functional psychoses of late onset, *Eur Arch Psychiatry* (1997) 247:176–89.

Herbert M, Jacobson S, Late paraphrenia, *Br J Psychiatry* (1967) 113:461–9.

Howard R, Almeida O, Levy R, Phenomenology, demography and diagnosis in late paraphrenia, *Psychol Med* (1994) 24:397–410.

Howard R, Castle D, O'Brien J et al, Permeable walls, floors, ceilings and doors. Partition delusions in late paraphrenia, *Int J Geriatr Psychiatry* (1992) 7:719–24.

Jeste D, Harris M, Krull A et al, Clinical and neuropsychological characteristics of patients with late-onset schizophrenia, *Am J Psychiatry* (1995) 152:722–30.

Jeste D, Harris M, Pearlson G et al, Late-onset schizophrenia: studying clinical validity, *Psychiatr Clin North Am* (1988) 11:1–13.

Kay D, Roth M, Environmental and hereditary factors in the schizophrenias of old age ('late paraphrenia') and their bearing on the general problem of causation in schizophrenia, *J Ment Sci* (1961) 107:649–86.

Leuchter A, Spar JE, The late-onset psychoses, *J Nerv Ment Dis* (1985) 173:488–94.

Liddle P, Barnes T, Syndromes of chronic schizophrenia, *Br J Psychiatry* (1990) 157:558–61.

McGlashan TH, The Chestnut Lodge follow-up study: II. Long-term outcome of schizophrenia and the affective disorders, *Arch Gen Psychiatry* (1984) 41:586–601.

McGlashan TH, A selective review of recent North American long-term followup studies of schizophrenia, *Schizophr Bull* (1988) 14:515–41.

McGorry P, Paradigm failure in functional psychosis: review and implications, *Aust N Z J Psychiatry* (1991) 25:43–55.

Mulsant B, Stergoiu A, Keshavan M et al, Schizophrenia in late life: elderly patients admitted to an acute care psychiatric hospital, *Schizophr Bull* (1993) 19:709–21.

Naguib M, Levy R, Late paraphrenia: neuropsychological impairment and structural brain abnormalities on computed tomography, *Int J Geriatr Psychiatry* (1987) 2:83–90.

Paskavitz JF, Lippa CF, Hamos JE et al, Role of the dorsomedial nucleus of the thalamus in Alzheimer's disease, *J Geriatr Psychiatry Neurol* (1995) 8:32–7.

Pearlson G, Dreger L, Rabins P et al, A chart review study of late-onset and early-onset schizophrenia, *Am J Psychiatry* (1989) 146:1568–74.

Post F, *Persistent Persecutory States of the Elderly* (Permagon Press: Oxford, 1966).

Roth M, The natural history of mental disorder in old age, *J Ment Sci* (1955) 101:281–301.

Rowan E, Phantom boarders as a symptom of late paraphrenia, *Am J Psychiatry* (1984) 141:580–1.

Sachdev P, Brodaty H, Rose N et al, Schizophrenia with onset after age 50 years: neurological, neuropsychological and MRI investigation, *Br J Psychiatry* (1999) 175:416–21.

Tsuang M, Lyons M, Faraone S, Heterogeneity of schizophrenia: conceptual models and analytic strategies, *Br J Psychiatry* (1990) **156**:17–26.

Van Os J, Howard R, Takei N et al, Increasing age is a risk factor for psychosis in the elderly, *Soc Psychiatry Psychiatr Epidemiol* (1995) 30:161–4.

Yassa R, Suranyi-Cadotte B, Clinical characteristics of late-onset schizophrenia and delusional disorder, *Schizophr Bull* (1993) 19:701–7.

Part I

Late-onset schizophrenia

chapter 3

Epidemiology of late-onset schizophrenia

David J. Castle

The phenomenology and nosology of late-onset schizophrenia has been outlined in Chapter 1 of this volume, and will not be reiterated here. Suffice to say that the first manifestation of a nonaffective nonorganic psychotic illness in late- and very-late life is a clinical reality. Table 3.1 outlines how such cases

Table 3.1 A comparison of early- and very-late-onset schizophrenia

Parameter	Early-onset	Very-late-onset (>60 years)
Gender	Males > females (especially childhood onset)	Females >> males
Phenomenology	Positive, negative, and disorganized symptoms all seen. Negative symptoms often prominent. Formal thought disorder common	Florid persecutory delusions; prominent hallucinations; negative symptoms and formal thought disorder are rare
Premorbid functioning	Impairment across multiple domains, including social and educational	Poor social adjustment common, but premorbid occupational functioning usually unimpaired
Longitudinal course	Poor social and occupational outcome	Good preservation of affect and personality. Social outcome often impaired; few progress to dementia
Response to antipsychotic medication	Positive symptoms respond but often partially. Treatment resistance common	Positive symptoms usually respond

From Orr and Castle (2003); reproduced with permission.

contrast with early-onset schizophrenia patients. This chapter concentrates on the epidemiology of late-onset nonaffective nonorganic psychotic disorders, excluding delusional (paranoid) disorders.

Methodological issues

The epidemiology of late-onset schizophrenia is an area beset by methodological problems, as articulated elsewhere (Castle, 1999). These problems include:

- Changing conceptualizations of what constitutes 'late-onset', with arbitrary age-at-onset cut-off points being applied according to different sets of diagnostic criteria – for example, 45 years in DSM-III (American Psychiatric Association, 1980) and 60 years according to Roth (1955).
- Variable age cut-offs being applied in population-based studies of psychotic disorders; for example, 54 years in the World Health Organization's 'Determinants of Outcome of Severe Mental Illness' study (Jablensky et al, 1992); 59 years in the Mannheim (Germany) 'ABC' study (Häfner et al, 1993); and 64 years in the Australian 'Study of Low Prevalence Disorders' (Jablensky et al, 2000).
- Changing nomenclature; for example, Kraepelin's (1919) 'dementia praecox' and 'paraphrenia', Bleuler's (1911) 'group of schizophrenias', Roth's (1955) 'late paraphrenia', Post's (1966) 'persistent persecutory states in the elderly', and the International Late-Onset Schizophrenia Group's consensus terms, 'late-onset schizophrenia' and 'very-late-onset schizophrenia-like psychosis' (Howard et al, 2000) (see Chapter 1).
- Variations in sets of diagnostic criteria used to diagnose schizophrenia; for example, the very stringent diagnostic criteria of Feighner et al (1972) essentially biased samples towards early-onset severe forms of schizophrenia.
- Lack of consistent application of standardized diagnostic questionnaires in clinical or population-based studies (e.g. Parsons, 1964; Williamson et al, 1964).
- Heterogeneity among clinical samples, with co-aggregation of some 'organic' cases (Holden, 1987).
- Different sampling frames; for example, the general population (e.g. Parsons, 1964; Williamson et al, 1964), all mental health contacts (e.g.

Castle and Murray, 1993), or mental health hospital admissions (e.g. Van Os et al, 1995).

These issues make interpretation of the literature on late-onset schizophrenia difficult, to say the least. Here, in an attempt to simplify matters, I have selectively reviewed studies of schizophrenia or 'schizophrenia-like psychosis' that have included cases over the age of 40, but have concentrated on those with an onset after the age of 60, as these might be considered a relatively discrete group (Howard et al, 2000). Following the general guidelines of the 'International Late-Onset Schizophrenia Group' (Howard et al, 2000), I have made a distinction, where possible, between patients with an onset between 40 and 60 years of age ('late-onset schizophrenia') and those over 60 years (here I have reverted to Roth's [1955] term 'late paraphrenia').

Prevalence studies

Early prevalence studies attempted to determine 'cases' in the general population, essentially by ascertaining all residents of a defined residential area who met criteria for a late-onset psychotic disorder. Thus, Parsons (1964), in a study in a Welsh town, reported a prevalence of late paraphrenia of 1.7% of persons over the age of 65, while a Scottish study published the same year (Williamson et al, 1964) found the rate to be around 1% of elderly people. Problems with these early studies include the lack of validated diagnostic questionnaires; the failure to apply stringent sets of diagnostic criteria, with careful exclusion of 'organic' cases; and the fact that one would expect paranoid individuals to be selectively unlikely to wish to participate in any such survey.

More recent and methodologically more robust studies include a study of 612 community-living Chinese over age 65, living in Singapore (Kua, 1992). Using the GMS-AGECAT criteria, the rate for schizophrenia/paranoia was 0.5%. In contrast, a much larger study in the UK (Copeland et al, 1998), using a sample of 5222 people over age 64 ascertained as part of the MRC-ALPHA (Ageing in Liverpool-Health Aspects) study, found a rate of GMS-AGECAT-defined schizophrenia of only 0.12% (95% CI 0.04–0.25).

In the large-scale Epidemiological Catchment Area (ECA) survey of psychopathology in the United States general population, the reported 1-year prevalence rates for schizophrenia were 0.6% for people aged between 45 and 64, and 0.2% for those over 65 years (Keith et al, 1991). However, this study relied on lay-administered interviews using the Diagnostic Interview Schedule (DIS), which has been criticized on the basis of validity. Perhaps more interesting than diagnostic prevalence rates are the reported rates of 'psychotic' phenomena among elderly people surveyed. Thus, using the Epidemiological Catchment Area (ECA) data, Tien (1991) showed rates of visual hallucinosis of around 20 per 1000 in males and 18 per 1000 in females across the adult life-span, with a steep rise in the later years of life. These data lend some insight into the interaction of age with the manifestation of psychotic phenomena.

Another approach to the prevalence problem is to determine, among samples of patients with a diagnosis of 'schizophrenia', what proportion have a late onset of illness. Harris and Jeste (1988) reviewed the literature then available on this topic, and computed weighted means (weighting according to sample size) such that around 23.5% of cases had an onset after the age of 40. Turning their attention to those samples specifically of late-onset patients (mostly over the age of 40), means were 57.5% in the fifth decade, 30.2% in the sixth, and 12.3% over the age of 60. This equates to overall proportions of all schizophrenia patients of 13%, 7%, and 3%, respectively.

Incidence studies

Incidence studies (i.e. assessing the number of new cases manifesting the illness for the first time over a defined period) are far more difficult to conduct, as they require ongoing case finding. Also, as noted above, many of the large population-based schizophrenia studies simply excluded late-onset cases. Furthermore, schizophrenia at any age, let alone with onset in old age, is a rare occurrence, and this militates either very large sampling frames or protracted periods of case ascertainment to accumulate statistically meaningful data. This is evidenced by the MRC-ALPHA study of Copeland and colleagues (see above), which reported 95% confidence limits for incidence rates for schizophrenia and delusional disorder after age 65 to be 0.00 to 110.70 per 100,000 population per year, making any estimate of a 'true' rate impossible.

Thus, the only feasible way of determining incidence rates for late-onset schizophrenia is to use case register or hospitalization data. This approach has the drawback, of course, that not all 'cases' seek help, a point underlined by the community-based study of Christenson and Blazer (1984) in the United States, which found that, of the individuals who exhibited paranoid ideation, only half felt the need for professional help; even fewer had actually accessed such help. Also, many people whose onset of schizophrenia is in late life have good occupational functioning in the setting of long-standing social isolation (see below), suggesting that they would not be likely to come to the attention of health professionals, either directly or through family and friends. Thus, administrative data are almost inevitably biased and under-representative of all cases in the community.

Hospital admission and case registers also tend to rely on administrative diagnoses, which may be inaccurate. The sample reported by Castle and Murray (1993) is one of the few to actually re-diagnose all potential cases of schizophrenia and related disorders, across all ages of onset, and according to a range of different diagnostic criteria. This study used the Camberwell Cumulative Psychiatric Case Register, which recorded all contacts with the psychiatric services of South-East London (UK) (not just admissions) over a period of 20 years from the mid-1960s. All available material was used to re-diagnose cases, using the Operational Criteria Checklist for Psychotic Disorders (OPCRIT) (McGuffin et al, 1991). Overall, 12% of cases had their first onset of illness after age 60. Of interest was that a high proportion of cases with a broad ICD-9 (WHO, 1980) diagnosis of schizophrenia or related disorders (including 'late paraphrenia'), met stringent criteria for schizophrenia as defined by the American Psychiatric Association in the revised version of DSM-III, the DSM-IIIR (American Psychiatric Association, 1987). Thus, 56% of patients with an onset after 60 met DSM-IIIR criteria for schizophrenia, versus 37% of those individuals with an onset before age 25 (Castle et al, 1998). This underscores the fact that many late-onset cases have florid and often bizarre psychotic symptoms, often in conjunction with hallucinations.

Van Os and colleagues (1995) took a somewhat different approach to the problem of the impact of age on risk for the first manifestation of schizophrenia. They used hospital admission data to show that the risk of schizophrenia actually increased with age, on average 11% per 5-year period over the age of 60.

Gender differences

It is usually reported that, over the full lifespan, schizophrenia tends to affect males and females at roughly equal rates. This overall finding does not do justice to the complexity of differences in risk for schizophrenia between the sexes. As we (Castle, 1999) have shown in the Camberwell Register study (see above), the age-at-onset distributions differ markedly between the sexes (see Figure 3.1). Thus, reliance on means and differences between mean ages at

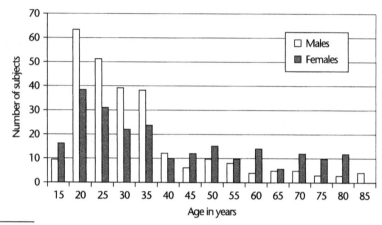

Figure 3.1 *Age at onset distribution, males and females. Reproduced from Castle (1999), with permission.*

onset between men and women simply does not make sense, as the distributions are not normally distributed. Being cognizant of the complexity of the
onset-age differentials between men and women might usefully inform our
understanding of risk factors for the group of disorders we commonly sub-
sume under the label 'schizophrenia' (see Castle and Murray, 1993).

There is no doubt that women are at greater risk for the first onset of a
schizophrenia-like psychosis in late life than men. Table 3.2 shows a selection
of studies, from different settings and using different definitions of schizophrenia and related disorders, selected from the literature spanning a period
of over 30 years. The excess of females among late-onset cases is not simply a
reflection of the relative longevity of women. Rather, it suggests a particular
vulnerability of women to the first onset of a paranoid psychosis in late life.
Presumably this has to do with differential aging effects on the female brain,
compared with that of the male. For example, a possible contributory factor
is the differential rate of loss of dopamine D2 receptors between the sexes,
with males losing D2 receptors at a faster rate than women, such that in late
life women have a relative excess of such receptors (see Castle, 1999).

Risk factors

The most robust risk factor for late-onset schizophrenia, as in early-onset
cases, is genetic. It also appears that generally the familial risk for schizophrenia among late-onset cases is lower than for early-onset cases, despite the

Table 3.2 Selected series of late-onset schizophrenia patients reporting gender ratio

Reference	Number of cases	Ascertainment method	Diagnosis	Age (years)	Ratio female:male
Kay (1963)	57	Hospital admissions	Late paraphrenia*	>60	5.3:1
Herbert & Jacobsen (1967)	47	Hospital admissions	Systematized delusion ± hallucinations; not demented	>65	22.5:1
Huber et al (1975)	644	Hospital admissions	Late-onset schizophrenia; nonorganic	>40	1.8:1
Bland (1977)	6064	First admissions	ICD-8 schizophrenia	>40	1.6:1
Blessed & Wilson (1982)	320	Hospital admissions	Late paraphrenia*	>65	6:1
Grahame (1984)	25	Consecutive referrals	Late paraphrenia*	>60	3.2:1
Rabins et al (1984)	35	Hospital admissions	Persistent delusional state; absence of mood or cognitive disorder	>44	10.7:1
Jørgensen & Munk-Jørgensen (1985)	106	First admissions	ICD-8 schizophrenia, paranoid state, reactive psychosis, other psychoses	>60	2.2:1
Holden (1987)	37	Case register	Late paraphrenia* (13 cases considered 'organic' at follow-up)	>60 >44	7:1 to 3:1† 2.3:1
Castle & Murray (1993)	477	Case register	ICD-9 schizophrenia and related disorders, paraphrenia, atypical psychoses	>60	4.4:1
Almeida et al (1995)	47	Referrals from a number of psychiatric settings	Late paraphrenia*	>65	9:1

* Akin to Roth's (1955) criteria.
† Dependent on whether 'organic' cases are included.
From Castle (1999), reproduced with permission.

fact that female schizophrenia patients are overall more likely than their male counterparts to have such a genetic loading. However, this area is bedeviled by methodological problems, including problems of case ascertainment among relatives who might have died either before the conduct of the study, or at least before going through the entire period of risk for a schizophrenia-like illness (should late-onset 'breed true'). In one of the few well-conducted family history studies of late paraphrenia cases that included matched controls, Howard et al (1997) found no significant increase in family loading for schizophrenia, but did show an excess of family members with depression, relative to normal controls. This suggests genetic heterogeneity among patients with late-onset schizophrenia.

Other risk factors for late-onset schizophrenia, relative to those for early-onset disorder, are shown in Table 3.3. Of these, one of the most extensively studied is sensory impairment, with a number of early studies suggesting an over-representation of both auditory and (to a lesser extent) visual impairment in such patients. However, an interesting twist to the tale lies in the findings of Prager and Jeste (1993) who, in a careful study of patients with late-onset schizophrenia, reported an excess of uncorrected, but not corrected, sensory impairment. This suggests that help-seeking behavior might play a part in earlier association findings.

People with late-onset schizophrenia tend to be socially isolated, but it is difficult to be sure whether this is causal or related to the illness itself, as paranoid ideation would tend to lead people to avoid socializing. Also, people who manifest schizophrenia in late life have often been socially impaired throughout their lives, and are thus less likely than their age-related peers to be married and to have a social network. Of interest in their premorbid history is that in general people with late-onset schizophrenia have good occupational functioning, which is in contrast to their lack of social connectedness, and also differs from early-onset cases (see Table 3.3).

Other factors associated with early-onset schizophrenia, notably neurodevelopmental markers such as obstetric complications, have not been extensively studied in late-onset cases. Castle et al (1997) used the Camberwell Register sample to compare such risks in early- and late-onset cases, and found significantly higher rates of obstetric complications in the early-onset group (14.1% vs 4.5% in those with late onset; relative risk 0.29; 95% CI 0.03–2.29). However, this was a case record study, and thus almost certainly underestimated rates of such risk factors.

Table 3.3 Putative risk factors for early- and very-late-onset schizophrenia

Putative risk factor	Early-onset	Very-late-onset (>60 years)
Genetic	+ + FH schizophrenia	+ FH schizophrenia + FH depression in some studies
Sensory impairment		+ Expressly unadjusted visual and hearing
Social isolation	+ Often consequent upon prodrome or illness itself	+ + Often antedates illness onset
Premorbid personality	Shy/withdrawn; schizotypal	+ Paranoid/schizoid traits
Pregnancy and birth complications	+ Associated with early onset, expressly in males*; limited data in childhood onset	No unequivocal evidence of an association
Structural brain abnormalities	+ + Gray matter reduction, generally considered to antedate illness onset; some evidence of progressive changes*	+ Gray matter volume reduction, similar to those in early-onset schizophrenia
Neurocognitive impairment	Diffuse impairment; possibly more pronounced in attention, memory, and executive function*	Diffuse impairment; nonspecific*

FH, family history; +, positive; + +, strong positive. *Denotes that findings are based on very few studies.
From Orr and Castle (2003), reproduced with permission.

Conclusions

This chapter has outlined the epidemiology of late-onset schizophrenia, covering prevalence and incidence studies, and studies that have assessed risk factors. Some of the inconsistencies in the literature can be explained in terms of methodological problems, although it is increasingly apparent that late-onset cases (as those with an early onset of illness) are a heterogeneous group with variable manifestations and consequent upon variable constellations of risk factors, often working in conjunction with normal aging processes. Some insights into such processes are provided by neuroimaging and neuropsychological studies in such patients; these issues are addressed in Chapters 4 and 5 of this book.

References

Almeida OP, Howard RJ, Levy R, David AS, Cognitive and clinical diversity in psychotic states arising in late life (late paraphrenia), *Psychol Med* (1995) 25:699–714.

American Psychiatric Association, *Diagnostic and Statistical Manual of Mental Disorders*, 3rd edn (DSM-III) (American Psychiatric Association: Washington, DC, 1980).

American Psychiatric Association, *Diagnostic and Statistical Manual of Mental Disorders*, 3rd edn (revised) (DSM-IIIR) (American Psychiatric Association: Washington, DC, 1987).

Bland RC, Demographic aspects of functional psychoses in Canada, *Acta Psychiatr Scand* (1997) 55:369–80.

Blessed G, Wilson ID, The contemporary natural history of mental disorder in old age, *Br J Psychiatry* (1982) 141:59–67.

Bleuler E, Die spatschizophrenen Krankheitsbilder (The clinical picture in late schizophrenia), *Fortschr Neurol Psyuchiatr* (1911) 15:259–90.

Castle DJ, Gender and age at onset in schizophrenia. In: Howard R, Rabins P, Castle DJ, eds, *Late Onset Schizophrenia* (Wrightson Biomedical: Hampshire, UK, 1999) 147–64.

Castle DJ, Murray RM, The epidemiology of late onset schizophrenia, *Schizophr Bull* (1993) 19:691–9.

Castle DJ, Wessely S, Howard R, Murray RM, Schizophrenia with onset at the extremes of adult life, *Int J Geriatr Psychiatry* (1997) 12:712–17.

Castle DJ, Wessely S, Van Os J, Murray RM, *Psychosis in the Inner City: The Camberwell First Episode Study* (Psychology Press: Hove, 1998).

Christenson R, Blazer D, Epidemiology of persecutory ideation in an elderly population in the community, *Am J Psychiatry* (1984) 141:59–67.

Copeland JRM, Davidson ME, Scott A et al, Schizophrenia and delusional disorder in old age: community prevalence, incidence and three-year outcome in Liverpool, *Schizophr Bull* (1998) 24:153–61.

Feighner JP, Robins E, Guze SB et al, Diagnostic criteria for use in psychiatric research, *Arch Gen Psychiatry* (1972) 26:57–63.

Grahame PS, Schizophrenia in old age (late paraphrenia), *Br J Psychiatry* (1984) 145:493–95.

Häfner H, Riecher-Rössler A, an der Heiden W et al, Generating and testing a causal explanation of the gender difference at first onset of schizophrenia, *Psychol Med* (1993) 23:925–40.

Harris MJ, Jeste DV, Late-onset schizophrenia: an overview, *Schizophr Bull* (1988) 14:39–55.

Herbert ME, Jacobsen S, Late paraphrenia, *Br J Psychiatry* (1967) 113:461–9.

Holden NL, Late paraphrenia or the paraphrenias? A descriptive study with 10-year follow-up, *Br J Psychiatry* (1987) 150:635–9.

Howard R, Graham C, Sham P et al, A controlled family study of late-onset non-affective psychosis (late paraphrenia), *Br J Psychiatry* (1997) 170:511–14.

Howard R, Rabins PV, Seeman MV, for the International Late-Onset Schizophrenia Group. Late-onset schizophrenia and very-late-onset schizophrenia-like psychosis: an international consensus, *Am J Psychiatry* (2000) 157:172–8.

Huber G, Gross G, Schüttler R, Spätschizophrenie, *Arch Psychiatr Nervenkr* (1975) 221:53–66.

Jablensky A, McGrath J, Herrman H et al, Psychotic disorders in urban areas: an overview of the Study of Low Prevalence Disorders, *Aust N Z J Psychiatry*, (2000) 34:221–36.

Jablensky A, Sartorius N, Ernberg G et al, *Schizophrenia: Manifestations, Incidence and Course in Different Countries; A World Health Organization Ten-Country Study.*

Psychological medicine Monograph, Vol. 20. (Cambridge University Press: Cambridge, 1992) 1–97.

Jørgensen P, Munk-Jørgensen P, Paranoid psychoses in the elderly, *Acta Psychiatr Scand* (1985) **72**:358–63.

Kay DWK, Late paraphrenia and its bearning on the aetiology of schizophrenia, *Acta Psychiatr Scand* (1963) **39**:159–69.

Keith SJ, Regier DA, Rae DS, Schizophrenic disorders. In: Robins LN, Regier DA, eds, *Psychiatric Disorders in America* (New York: Free Press, 1991).

Kraepelin E, *Dementia Praecox and Paraphrenia* (E & S Livingstone: Edinburgh, 1919).

Kua EHA, Community study of mental disorders in elderly Singaporean Chinese using the GMS-AGECAT package, *Aust N Z J Psychiatry*, (1992) **26**:502–6.

McGuffin P, Farmer AE, Harcey I, A polydiagnostic application of operational criteria in studies of psychotic illness: development and reliability of the OPCRIT system, *Arch Gen Psychiatry* (1991) **48**:764–70.

Orr KDG, Castle DJ, Schizophrenia at the extremes of life. In: Murray RM, Jones PB, Susser E et al, eds, *The Epidemiology of Schizophrenia* (Cambridge University Press: Cambridge, 2003) 167–90.

Parsons PL, Mental health of Swansea's old folk, *Br J Preventative Social Med* (1964) **19**:43–7.

Post F. *Persistent Persecutory States in the Elderly* (Pergamon Press: Oxford, 1966).

Prager S, Jeste DV, Sensory impairment in late life schizophrenia, *Schizophr Bull* (1993) **19**:755–71.

Rabins P, Paulker S, Thomas J, Can schizophrenia begin after age 44?, *Compr Psychiatry* (1984) **25**:290–3.

Roth M, The natural history of mental disorder in old age, *J Mental Sci* (1955) **101**:281–301.

Tien AY, Distribution of hallucinations in the population, *Soc Psychiatry Psychiatr Epidemiol* (1991) **26**:287–92.

Van Os J, Howard R, Takei N et al, Increasing age is a risk factor for psychosis in the elderly, *Soc Psychiatry Psychiatr Epidemiol* (1995) **30**:161–4.

Williamson J, Stokoe IH, Gray S et al, Old people at home: their unreported needs, *Lancet* (1964) **I**:1117–20.

World Health Organization, *International Classification of Diseases*, 9th revision (ICD-9) (World Health Organization: Geneva, 1980).

chapter 4

Neuroimaging in late-onset schizophrenia

Mark Walterfang, Ramon Mocellin, Dennis Velakoulis and Christos Pantelis

Introduction

The majority of neuroimaging studies investigating structural and functional imaging abnormalities in schizophrenia have examined early-onset illness beginning in adolescence or young adulthood (Liddle and Pantelis, 2003). An aging population in developed countries, particularly beyond the seventh decade, has focused interest on psychosis with onset in middle age or beyond. Research into a later-onset group may expand our understanding of the structural and functional deficits of psychotic disorders and inform debate on the putative neurodevelopmental models of schizophrenia (Palmer et al, 1999; Velakoulis et al, 2000; Pantelis et al, 2003b).

Schizophrenia-like psychosis in older and younger patients can result from a variety of medical and neurological conditions, including neoplasia, trauma, infections, and degenerative diseases (Lewis, 1995). Psychotic symptoms can also be manifestations of other psychiatric conditions, such as affective disorders. There is consensus, however, that schizophrenia with onset later in life is a discrete clinical entity (Howard et al, 2000).

Presentations of schizophrenia later in life have been divided into a late-onset schizophrenia (LOS) group (onset 40–60 years), and a very-late-onset schizophrenia-like psychosis (VLOSLP) (onset after 60 years) (Howard et al, 2000), which is similar to patients previously described as having late-onset paranoid psychoses (Riecher-Rössler et al, 2003). It has been argued that these patient groups cannot truly be called 'schizophrenia' as patients with early-onset schizophrenia (EOS) differ not only in age of onset but in clinical features, course, neuropathology and neuroimaging findings and the diagnosis itself implies an illness of neurodevelopmental origin (Andreasen, 1999).

These difficulties with categorical definition complicate studies comparing people with LOS with other patient groups or controls on clinical, pathological or neuroimaging measures. Additionally, the finding of an increased rate of neuroimaging abnormalities in the otherwise healthy aging population (Christiansen et al, 1994; Grossman et al, 1997) and the diverse nature of brain lesions that may produce psychotic symptoms in the elderly (Lewis, 1995) further complicates the differentiation of clinically relevant and irrelevant neuroimaging findings in this patient population. Finally, comparing the small number of studies examining neuroimaging correlates of LOS is rendered difficult because of differences in image acquisition, analysis and study methodology in addition to differences in study population (Jani et al, 2000).

Neuroimaging techniques traditionally have been categorized into those defining brain anatomy and those attempting to define brain function. This paradigm has become less distinct with technological advances and combinations of techniques, such as co-analysis of structural and functional magnetic resonance imaging, although it remains the simplest means to describe the 'division of labor' in neuroimaging.

Structural brain abnormalities were first described by pneumoencephalogram (PEG) analysis of patients with psychiatric illnesses in the1930s (Rabins et al, 2000). Greater delineation of brain structures followed the development of computed tomography (CT) in the 1970s (Ambrose and Hounsfield, 1973). The advent of magnetic resonance imaging (MRI) enabled the production of brain images with highly resolved anatomical detail, particularly in gray matter structures (Lock et al, 1990). Further development of MR principles with developments such as diffusion tension imaging (DTI) that delineate white matter tracts, allowing assessment of anatomical connectivity, hold a great deal of promise in uniting anatomic and functional pathology in psychiatric illness (Taylor et al, 2004).

Functional neuroimaging had its origins in the 1970s with the development of positron emission tomography (PET) (Parsey and Mann, 2003) and subsequently single photon emission computed tomography (SPECT), where regional blood flow and glucose metabolism provide an index of regional brain function (Vasile, 1996). Newer imaging techniques to examine brain metabolism have evolved out of MRI in the last decade. Functional MRI (fMRI) measures deoxyhemoglobin concentration and thus co-analyses anatomic structure and oxidative metabolism (Jezzard and Song, 1996). Magnetic resonance spectroscopy (MRS) examines the spectra produced by common organic compounds in a magnetic field to measure specific metabolite levels in different white and gray matter regions (Malhi et al, 2002). Another technique, magnetoencephalography (MEG) can characterize brain electrical activity – a further index of function – by measuring magnetic fields emanating from the cortex as a result of surface electrical currents (Reite et al, 1996).

This chapter outlines the major findings of studies using structural and functional neuroimaging to study LOS. We also describe the limitations and methodological difficulties of such studies as well as where the future of research in this field may lie.

Structural neuroimaging

PEG studies in the 1930s were the first to demonstrate ventricular and sulcal enlargement in younger patients with schizophrenia (Haug, 1965). As CT and MRI became available, these findings were confirmed (Liddle and Pantelis, 2003), and indicated that these changes were due to an increased ventricle to brain ratio (VBR), reflecting regional volume loss in frontal and temporal zones (Dennert and Andreasen, 1983; Shenton et al, 2001). Although fewer in number, studies examining global and regional volumes have also been undertaken in LOS.

Computed tomography

The majority of CT studies have demonstrated increased VBR in patients with later-onset schizophrenia (Naguib and Levy, 1987; Rabins et al, 1987; Burns et al, 1989), while two studies have failed to find a difference in VBR (Howard et al, 1992; Barak et al, 2002). Additionally, these studies have identified that the degree of VBR increase was not as pronounced as in patients with Alzheimer's disease and psychosis (Rabins et al, 1987) and that those patients with more significant change did not differ in clinical or neuropsychological presentation (Naguib and Levy, 1987).

CT studies of cortical volumes have shown that patients without first-rank symptoms (FRS) showed greater cortical atrophy than those with FRS, supporting Trimble's notion that FRS reflect greater dominant temporal cortical changes (Trimble, 1990). In a study of VLOSLP compared with age-matched EOS, Barak et al (2002) found that the VLOSLP group had greater cerebellar VBR but not frontal VBR, and no difference in degree of atrophy or periventricular leukoencephalopathy. White matter changes in late-onset psychosis have been reported in two case series studies by Miller et al, which found that three of five patients (Miller et al, 1986), and five of 27 patients with late-onset psychosis showed extensive white matter disease. The latter study did not identify any white matter changes in any of 60 age-matched controls (Miller et al, 1989). However, these studies did not exclude patients with cerebrovascular disease including cortical and subcortical infarction.

In summary, increased VBR compared with controls is the most robust CT-based finding, shown in all but one study. The small number of studies and the lack of other structural measures make it difficult to interpret the relationship of clinical variables to CT-based structural measures.

MRI

Ventricle to brain ratio/ventricular volumes

The improved definition and volumetric sensitivity of MRI has not entirely replicated the findings of increased (ventricle to brain ratio) VBR in LOS, and studies using MRI have tended to focus on individual volumes as these are likely a more sensitive measure than changes to the ventricular system (Arndt et al, 1991; Woods et al, 1991).

A number of studies have identified increased VBR in patients with LOS compared with control subjects (Pearlson et al, 1993; Howard et al, 1994; Corey-Bloom et al, 1995; Barta et al, 1997; Sachdev et al, 1999a; Rabins et al, 2000), although negative findings have been described (Miller et al, 1991). Comparison to other patient groups has shown that the ventricular changes are not as great as those found in patients with Alzheimer's disease (AD) (Rabins et al, 1987; Barta et al, 1997) but are greater than in patients with late-onset affective disorders (Rabins et al, 2000) and equal to changes in age-matched patients with EOS (Corey-Bloom et al, 1995; Sachdev et al, 1999a).

Howard et al (1994) divided a cohort of LOS patients into ICD-10 diagnostic groups, and found that LOS patients only had subtly increased volumes compared to controls, whereas patients with delusional disorder showed much greater volumetric change. The single study that has compared LOS patients with late-onset depression/bipolar patients and controls found that LOS patients had third ventricular and right temporal horn enlargement but no change in cortical volume, whereas the converse applied for both affective disorder groups, suggesting that the neuropathologies of these disorders in senescence are divergent (Rabins et al, 2000).

Increased ventricular size has been thought to reflect cortical atrophy, but this relationship is controversial. Early studies (e.g. Weinberger et al, 1979) that used CT scanning in EOS subjects tended to show a low correlation between cortical atrophy and ventricular enlargement, otherwise seen in healthy controls (Jacoby and Levy, 1980; Dolan et al, 1986), and this 'uncoupling' has also been seen in CT-based studies of LOS patients (Naguib and Levy, 1987; Burns et al, 1989).

The ability of MRI to allow better delineation of regional brain volumes in EOS studies has provided further evidence that regional ventricular change reflects focal gray matter loss in the temporal lobes (Chance et al, 2002) and in the thalamus and insula cortex (Gaser et al, 2004). Enlargement of the third ventricle in those with LOS may reflect disruptions to adjacent diencephalic structures, which are involved in limbic system functioning and cortico-subcortical feedback (Bornstein et al, 1992). Similarly, the findings of lateral ventricular change may reflect processes similar to those described in EOS.

Cortical volume

While a wealth of evidence in EOS is suggestive of regionalized gray matter loss, at the onset of illness and with disease progression (Shenton et al, 2001; Velakoulis et al, 2002; Liddle and Pantelis, 2003; Pantelis et al, 2003a), similar studies in LOS are less conclusive, principally because of the smaller number of such studies and the lack of consistency in the available studies with regard to patient populations, regions examined, and methods used.

The studies that have investigated cortical volumes in patients and control subjects have largely found no differences in cortical gray matter volumes (Corey-Bloom et al, 1995; Howard et al, 1995b; Symonds et al, 1997) but have identified some regional differences in temporal lobe structures (Barta et al, 1997; Sachdev et al, 1999a). In comparison with age-matched EOS patients, LOS patients have been shown to have larger thalami (Corey-Bloom et al, 1995), similar anterior temporal reductions (Sachdev et al, 1999a) and greater mid-parietal reductions (Sachdev et al, 1999a). The authors of the latter study rightly interpret their visually based rating findings with caution against manual tracing methods (Sachdev et al, 1999a). Barta et al (1997) showed reductions compared with controls in both LOS and Alzheimer's groups in amygdala, hippocampus, and enterorhinal cortex, but found that reductions in the right superior temporal gyrus (STG) were seen only in the LOS group. An earlier CT-based study suggesting cerebellar volume loss in LOS (Barak et al, 2002) was not replicated by Sachdev and Brodaty (1999a), who manually traced cerebellar volume. Furthermore, this latter study is the only study to look at corpus callosum volume in LOS, and found a nonsignificant trend to reduced mid-sagittal volume in both EOS and LOS patients.

In summary, compared with the large number of EOS studies which have assessed regional brain volumes in a number of brain structures, the LOS literature is strikingly lacking in such studies. In particular, given the findings of hippocampal volume reduction in EOS and AD, a comparison of hippocampal volumetry across LOS, EOS, and AD would seem warranted.

White matter hyperintensities

White matter hyperintensities (WMHs) are visible regions of increased signal intensity seen on CT or MRI and which represent a heterogeneous group of histopathologic findings. WMHs have been linked to perivascular pathology, myelin thinning, gliosis, edema, and vascular lesions (Braffman et al, 1988a, 1988b; Grafton et al, 1991). Combined magnetic resonance and neuropathological analysis of post-mortem tissue suggests that ischemic myelin loss, altered myelin density, and ependymal loss are responsible (Thomas et al, 2003) for WMHs. WMHs occur frequently in the elderly without psychiatric disorder with prevalence rates between 30% and 90% (Bradley et al, 1984; Awad et al, 1987), are associated with advancing age and vascular risk factors (Bondareff et al, 1990; Deicken et al, 1991), and are present in other disorders including unipolar and bipolar depression (Swayze et al, 1990; O'Brien et al, 1996) and vascular and Alzheimer's dementias (Fazekas et al, 1987; Hershey et al, 1987).

Although an association between WMHs and late-onset psychosis was noted in the CT era (Miller et al, 1986, 1989), the prevalence of these lesions in LOS was not systematically studied until the advent of MRI scanning. An example MRI scan in a LOS patient can be seen in Figure 4.1.

Eight studies have examined WMHs in LOS patients compared to a control group (Breitner et al, 1990; Lesser et al, 1992; Corey-Bloom et al, 1995; Howard et al, 1995a; Keshavan et al, 1996; Symonds et al, 1997; Sachdev et al, 1999a; Rivkin et al, 2000). Four of these studies found no difference in WMHs between LOS and control groups (Corey-Bloom et al, 1995; Howard et al, 1995a; Symonds et al, 1997; Rivkin et al, 2000), with three of these four studies also finding no difference between LOS, EOS, and control groups (Corey-Bloom et al, 1995; Symonds et al, 1997; Rivkin et al, 2000). Three of the eight studies found increased WMHs compared with a control group (Breitner et al, 1990; Keshavan et al, 1996; Sachdev et al, 1999a). One study found WMHs of greater than 5 cm^2 in six of 12 patients with late-onset psychosis, with a mean

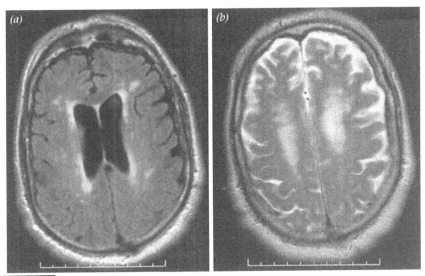

Figure 4.1 *Axial MRI scans of a 62-year-old male with first-presentation of a psychotic disorder. A T1-weighted image (a) demonstrates periventricular caps and rims, and scattered subcortical white matter hyperintensities. A T2-weighted image (b) at a higher axial slice shows extensive subcortical hyperintensities and anterior cortical sulcal widening.*

area six times greater in patients than in 100 age-matched controls (Lesser et al, 1992).

Methodological issues complicate the interpretation of these studies as a single body of work. The method of WMHs analysis ranges from visual scales (Breitner et al, 1990; Howard et al, 1995a; Keshavan et al, 1996; Sachdev et al, 1999a), interpretation of radiologists' written reports (Symonds et al, 1997), manual tracing (Tonkonogy and Geller, 1999), to no method described (Corey-Bloom et al, 1995). The patient samples also include patients with predominantly delusional disorder (Breitner et al, 1990), VLOSLP (Howard et al, 1995a) or no identification of the diagnostic breakdown of the LOS (Miller et al, 1989, 1991; Breitner et al, 1990).

The use of differing ordinal measures, usually in the form of visual rating scales, limits the conclusions that can be drawn from these early studies, although it has been suggested that visual rating scales (in the hands of trained and experienced raters) are more reliable than, and show moderate correlation with, manual tracing methods (Sachdev et al, 1999b). Studies using nominal measures lend themselves to a more rigorous statistical analysis. Sachdev and Brodaty (1999b) measured widths of 'rims' and 'caps' in periventricular regions and number of WMHs in other zones in LOS, EOS and control subjects, showing that LOS patients had greater volume of periventricular WMHs than either comparison group. The LOS patients in the study also demonstrated more hyperintensities in the thalamus than other subject groups, but no differences were seen in the basal ganglia or brainstem regions. This group also showed that WMH load correlated with verbal IQ, and with verbal memory and measures of intellectual function (Sachdev and Brodaty, 1999b). Rivkin et al (2000) manually traced and summed WMHs greater than one or two voxels in dimension to produce a nominal measure of WMH 'load' in 12 LOS, 10 EOS, and 28 control subjects, finding no significant difference between the groups – although 4 out of 5 patients with a WMH volume greater than 6 cm^3 were in the LOS group.

The role of white matter in psychotic disorders is being increasingly recognized (Bartzokis, 2002; Davis et al, 2003), and lesions of white matter structures could produce psychosis by affecting anatomical connectivity between regions to disrupt the functional synchrony upon which normal cognition, perception, and judgment depend. The significance of WMHs in elderly populations is unclear, as they are likely present to a small degree in most individuals beyond the age of 60 (Wen and Sachdev, 2004). In addition, WMHs visible on T2 images are likely not the best index of 'white matter load' as white matter which appears normal on conventional imaging may be abnormal on diffusion-weighted imaging (DWI), magnetization transfer imaging (MTI), T2-relaxometry (T2R), and magnetic resonance spectroscopy (MRS) in normal subjects (Firbank et al, 2003) and patients with demyelination (Leary et al, 1999; Kapellar et al, 2001; Whittal et al, 2002). Future studies exploring the role of WMHs in LOS would benefit from these MR sequences that may allow for more sensitive detection of white matter pathology.

Comparison to early-onset schizophrenia

The structural abnormalities reported in LOS have been described in EOS. These include enlarged global ventricular volume, lateral ventricles, and third but not fourth ventricle (Shelton et al, 1986; Shenton et al, 2001; Mark and Ulmer, 2004). In addition, the evidence of global cortical atrophy is similarly weak in EOS (Ward et al, 1996; Shenton et al, 2001), while evidence of abnormalities in the temporal lobe such as the superior temporal gyrus and amygdala are found regularly if not invariably (McCarley et al, 1999; Shenton et al, 2001; Liddle and Pantelis, 2003). However, some neurodevelopmental abnormalities reported with moderate frequency in EOS, such as cavum septum pellucidum, callosal dysgenesis, and abnormal gyrification have not been described in LOS (Almeida, 1999; McCarley et al, 1999). Volume reductions in the hippocampus have been robustly established in EOS (Nelson et al, 1998; Velakoulis et al, 1999), but only two studies in LOS have found conflicting findings (Howard et al, 1995b; Barta et al, 1997). This may be in some way due to the low base rate of neurodevelopmental abnormalities in both schizophrenic and control subject populations in combination with small sample sizes in most LOS studies, in addition to the dearth of studies examining specific medial temporal structures with volumetric methods.

When EOS and LOS groups have been compared with the same methodologies, results have shown more commonalities than differences – such as on measures of ventricular and sulcal size and regional cortical volumes (Pearlson et al, 1993; Sachdev et al, 1999a). Where the groups may diverge is on WMH measures, which have been found to be more prevalent and severe in LOS than EOS patients in most (Sachdev et al, 1999a, 1999b; Tonkonogy and Geller, 1999; Rivkin et al, 2000) but not all (Corey-Bloom et al, 1995; Symonds et al, 1997) studies. The significance of this is unclear, although it may be that the common abnormalities reflect shared heritable vulnerabilities to psychosis in both EOS and LOS (the 'first hit') that are impacted upon by temporally and neuropathologically disparate 'second hits' (such as intrauterine insult in EOS versus development of vascular white matter disease in LOS). Another possibility elaborated by Pearlson is that the 'second hit' in some LOS patients may merely be normal brain aging (Almeida, 1999), although this would be expected to affect both LOS and EOS patients equally when age-matched groups are compared.

Comparison to other psychiatric disorders

The findings reported in LOS, including those that are common to EOS, are not specific to either disorder. These include increased VBR, third ventricle enlargement, hippocampal volumetric reduction and elevated rate of WMHs, which are also seen in, for example, late-onset unipolar depression (Coffey et al, 1990; Rabins et al, 1991; O'Brien et al, 1996; Lloyd et al, 2004). Temporal lobe abnormalities in particular are also not disorder-specific, with hippocampal reductions reported in depression, bipolar disorder, and posttraumatic stress disorder (Gurvits et al, 1996; Velakoulis et al, 1999; Lloyd et al, 2004). In contrast, the STG abnormalities seen in LOS may be relatively specific to schizophrenia and differentiate it from other disorders (Velakoulis et al, 1999; Shenton et al, 2001). Alterations in ventricular size reflect changes in regional brain structures or abnormalities in the ventricular system itself, and hence are reported in a range of neurodegenerative diseases and hydro-cephalus (Shenton et al, 2001).

Studies that compare people with LOS to individuals with other disorders seen in this age group may point to some changes that differentiate between these disorders. Compared with Alzheimer's patients, LOS patients have less marked increases in VBR (Rabins et al, 1987; Pearlson et al, 1993; Barta et al, 1997) and third ventricle size (Pearlson et al, 1993). When cortical volumes are compared, they have comparable reductions in amygdala-hippocampal volumes without the global atrophy seen in AD, but greater volume loss in the STG (Barta et al, 1997). Rabins et al (2000) have also shown that late-onset affective disorder patients tend to demonstrate cortical atrophy, left sylvian fissure and bilateral temporal sulcal enlargement, while LOS subjects have enlarged third ventricles and right superior temporal horns. LOS may well then be differentiated from other late-life disorders by the regionally specific volumetric reductions in the STG and related CSF regions, and differentiated from EOS by a higher rate of WMHs in a subset of patients. However, the modest number of studies, their often small sample sizes (reflecting the difficulty in recruiting LOS patients without major confounding factors such as cerebrovascular disease), and methodological differences limit the conclusions that can be drawn about etiopathological mechanisms.

Functional neuroimaging

Positron emission tomography

Positron emission tomography (PET) is a technique for measuring the concentrations of positron-emitting radioisotopes within the tissue of living subjects, providing information on regional metabolism (using $[^{18}F]$-fluorodeoxyglucose) or blood flow (using $[^{15}O]$-water). In schizophrenic subjects, regional cerebral blood flow (rCBF) and neurotransmitter receptor density have been the most frequently studied (Soares and Innis, 1999).

EOS subjects differ from controls, demonstrating frontal hypometabolism at rest (Kim et al, 2000) and with psychological tasks such as those probing working memory (Berman et al, 1993). These types of studies are yet to be undertaken in LOS either at rest or with activation tasks. Given that neuropsychological deficits in LOS appear to mirror those in EOS to a significant degree, including in working memory (Almeida, 1999), comparing LOS patients with age-matched EOS patients or controls would be of interest.

Imaging of striatal dopamine D2 receptors using PET ligands such as [^{11}C]raclopride began in the 1980s, and provided a way to test the 'dopamine hypothesis' of schizophrenia. Many, but not all, studies have demonstrated (both in vivo and post mortem) increased levels of striatal D2 receptors in EOS, while extrastriatal D2 density has been rarely studied as D2 receptors exist in significantly lower levels at other sites (for a review, see Soares et al, 1999). In a study of 13 drug-naïve LOS patients with illness onset after the age of 55, Pearlson et al (1993) found similarly elevated levels of striatal D2 receptors compared to 17 unmatched controls when using [^{11}C]-methylspiperone as a dopamine receptor ligand. This is the only published study to date to confirm D2 elevation in LOS patients. Antipsychotic treatments are a major confound in such studies and there are no available studies of neuroleptic-naïve LOS patients. Further, unlike in the EOS field, there have been no PET studies to date examining extrastriatal dopamine, dopamine metabolism, and other neurotransmitter systems (such as serotonin) in LOS.

Single photon-emission computed tomography (SPECT)

SPECT utilizes photon-emitting radioisotopes to measure in vivo tissue metabolism and perfusion. In a similar fashion to PET, CT is used to produce an image of the organ or tissue under investigation. Brain SPECT has been used extensively in neurology for assistance with diagnosis and treatment planning for epilepsy and dementia, and in psychiatry it has been applied most to the study of schizophrenia (Camargo, 2001). Like PET, SPECT can be used to measure rCBF (usually using [^{99}Tc]-hexamethyl propyleneamine oxime, HMPAO) and can be combined with specific ligands that bind to particular receptor subtypes.

Mirroring PET findings, SPECT studies of EOS have demonstrated resting rCBF abnormalities such as hypofrontality (Krausz et al, 1996) and changes in rCBF with set shifting tasks (Berman et al, 1992). SPECT studies using the tracer [^{123}I]-iodobenzamide in EOS have shown exaggerated dopamine release to amphetamine challenge and increased resting occupancy of D2 receptors (for a review, see Abi-Dargham, 2004) but have not unequivocally shown increased striatal D2 receptors previously demonstrated using PET (Pilowsky et al, 1994).

Some workers have found similar resting rCBF changes in patients with LOS. In a group of 32 late-onset psychosis patients, 14 of whom met criteria for LOS, Lesser and colleagues (1992) used HMPAO in 20 of these patients (although the diagnostic breakdown is not reported) and blind raters to rate scans. The raters determined that 80% of patient scans showed frontotemporal hypoperfusion, whereas few of the 30 controls had any demonstrable reductions in perfusion (Lesser et al, 1993). Miller et al (1992) also used HMPAO in 45 patients with onset of psychosis after the age of 45 and compared their visual SPECT findings (again using blind raters) against 12 late-onset psychotic depression patients and 30 controls: 83% of both patient groups showed either frontal or temporal hypoperfusion compared with 27% of controls, although much higher rates of cerebrovascular disease were seen in both patient groups. An example SPECT demonstrating these changes can be seen in Figure 4.2.

In the most sophisticated functional imaging study in this patient population, Sachdev et al (1997) co-registered HMPAO-SPECT and volumetric MRI and manually traced regions of interest, finding reduced cortical perfusion in the frontal and temporal lobes bilaterally in 15 LOS patients compared with 27 controls. This was similar to perfusion patterns in an EOS group of seven subjects in the study, although temporal changes were more marked in LOS.

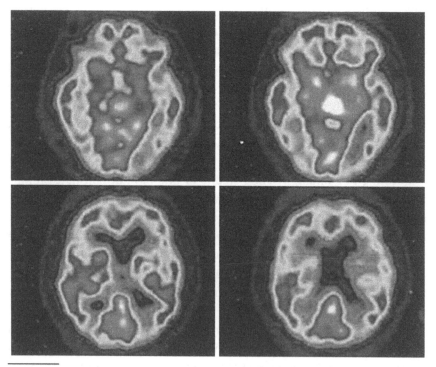

Figure 4.2 *HMPAO-SPECT scan in a 55-year-old male with first-episode psychosis. Note the patchy hypoperfusion, particularly in frontotemporal zones.*

Correlations of perfusion with MRI changes were generally low but basal ganglia perfusion correlated with basal ganglia hyperintensities on MRI in both patient groups. The authors concluded that there were few differences between LOS and EOS groups – with the LOS group not demonstrating significant evidence of coarse brain disease; here they diverge from earlier studies suggesting that hypoperfusion abnormalities may have been vascular in origin. No studies have yet examined the relationship to the predominant symptoms that characterize LOS.

In summary, although LOS cohorts may demonstrate evidence of increased cerebrovascular disease on SPECT, abnormalities of resting rCBF may be similar to those encountered in EOS, which mirrors much of the PET literature. More work is required to examine dopamine receptor activity and binding in striatal and extrastriatal regions in LOS, especially in antipsychotic-naïve patients, and to relate the findings to the symptoms in LOS. Such studies would go some way to determining if the underlying dopaminergic pathology is common to both early- and late-onset groups and to examining relationships to phenomenology.

MRS

MRS examines the MR-visible spectra of particular nuclei (such as ^{1}H or ^{31}P), allowing in vivo evaluation of brain neurochemistry via examination of frequency-signal intensity spectra which represent the metabolites or compounds that compose a targeted brain region (Malhi et al, 2002). Metabolites that can be measured include N-acetyl aspartate (NAA), choline, glucose, glutamate, membrane phospholipid metabolites such as phosophomonoesters (PME) and phosphodiesters (PDE) and markers of phosphate metabolism such as ATP (adenosine triphosphate).

Many MRS studies of EOS have demonstrated reduced levels of NAA and alterations to the NAA/creatine ratio in prefrontal cortical, temporal, hippocampal, and thalamic brain regions, suggestive of reductions in neuronal mass and integrity (Deicken et al, 2000; Vance et al, 2000). Additionally, alterations in PME and PDE have been repeatedly shown, suggesting abnormal neuronal membranes and/or abnormal neuronal breakdown (Vance et al, 2000). Although one group has found a negative correlation between the age of onset of EOS and hippocampal NAA/phosphocreatine measured by MRS (Delamillieure et al, 2002), studies with this very promising technique have not yet been undertaken in LOS patients.

Functional MRI

Functional MRI (fMRI) uses nuclear magnetic resonance principles to map local increases in blood flow and microvascular oxygenation, which reflect brain activation or metabolism. This can be reflected in the relative amount of deoxyhemoglobin in a given area, which in fMRI is described as a 'blood oxygenation level-dependent' (or 'BOLD') effect that can be observed by non-invasive MRI at high magnetic fields (Levin et al, 1995). Blood volume may also contribute to image contrast (Wishart et al, 2002). Resting blood volumes reflecting hypofrontality and decreased lateralization have been reported in a number of fMRI studies of EOS (Kindermann et al, 1997; Walter et al, 2003), as have reduction of activation with procedural learning (Kumari et al, 2002) and reduced hippocampal activation with word recognition tasks (Jessen et al, 2003), although most of these studies are small in number. As with other newly developed techniques, fMRI has not as yet been applied to the study of LOS.

Magnetoencephalography

Magnetoencephalography (MEG) measures extracranial magnetic fields, generated by intraneuronal ionic current flow in appropriately oriented cortical pyramidal cells. These very weak fields can be measured by detection coils, generating waveforms that can map electrical abnormalities with high accuracy and temporal resolution (Reite et al, 1999). MEG studies of schizophrenia have demonstrated a variety of findings including reductions in intrahemispheric asymmetry compared with controls (Reite et al, 1996) and possible cortical re-organization (Fehr et al, 2001). Unfortunately no MEG studies have been undertaken in LOS patients.

Conclusions

Definitional and categorical problems continue to complicate the study of LOS, particularly neuroimaging. Many early studies combined LOS, delusional disorder, affective psychosis, and psychotic disorder NOS groups into 'late-onset psychosis' cohorts, and very few studies of any kind have utilized the recent separation of LOS and VLOSLP groups.

Neuroimaging findings in LOS are, in general, similar to those seen in EOS. These include findings of increased VBR, regional temporal lobe reductions and similar patterns of resting blood flow, although these findings are not necessarily specific to schizophrenia. The role of WMHs in LOS remains unclear, although they may be of relevance in a subgroup of patients. Although the recent techniques of fMRI, MRS, and MEG have been employed extensively in the investigation of EOS, these methodologies have not been utilized in LOS. The lack of evidence for a specific pathologic process supports the view that schizophrenia-like psychoses in old age are likely to represent a syndrome with heterogeneous etiologies (Riecher-Rössler et al, 2003).

Future directions

Neuroimaging techniques have been developed to provide a noninvasive means to study brain structure and function. Although increasing anatomic detail has become evident, controversy regarding the pathologic correlates of common findings (such as WMHs) remains. Functional techniques have also been helpful, but heterogeneous findings have reinforced the complexity of brain structure–function relationships and it is difficult to disentangle this complexity in small heterogeneous samples. Future neuroimaging studies in LOS would benefit from improvements in patient selection (larger sample sizes, better separation of diagnostic groups, close matching of control or other patient groups) and a better understanding of the strengths and limitations of newer structural and functional imaging technologies.

Structural (MRI) and functional (SPECT, PET, MEG, EEG, fMRI) techniques have been combined to demonstrate functional deficits on a three-dimensional anatomic map. Combining techniques may make it possible to link anatomic abnormalities with functional deficits and patient symptoms to develop a better understanding of neuropsychiatric symptoms. With the advent of transcranial magnetic stimulation, it may be possible to image brain dysfunction and its response to treatment, and to modify treatment accordingly (Sack and Linden 2003). As many of these techniques are noninvasive it may also be possible to follow the clinical course of disorders such as LOS and develop neuroimaging correlates of clinical and functional progression.

Recent advances in imaging the human brain have brought neuroscience to a frontier where aspects of neuroanatomy, physiology, and chemistry have become increasingly integrated. A number of examples of such integration are emerging. Recent neuropathologic evidence has linked women with late onset of a schizophrenia-like psychosis to a restricted limbic tauopathy (Casanova et al, 2002). A recent study has also developed a technique of imaging beta-amyloid plaques in AD (Shoghi-Jadid et al, 2002). In the future it may be possible to utilize neuroimaging to measure and follow protein synthesis in the brain, including in response to treatment.

Although neuroimaging has advanced the understanding of neuropsychiatric illness considerably, many techniques have fallen short of their initial promise, such as in vivo receptor binding studies (Kumar, 2002). Further research integrating neuroimaging techniques with clinical findings and neuropathology is required to clarify the entity of late-onset psychosis. Further integration of these findings into clinical practice will remain a challenge for those involved in the care of this often vulnerable section of the community.

References

Abi-Dargham A, Do we still believe in the dopamine hypothesis? New studies bring new evidence, *Int J Neuropsychopharmacol* (2004) 7:S1–S5.

Almeida O, Neuropsychology of schizophrenia in late life. In: Howard R, Rabins PV, Castle DJ, eds, *Late Onset Schizophrenia* (Wrightson Biomedical Publishing: Petersfield, 1999).

Ambrose J, Hounsfield G, Computerised transverse axial tomography, *Br J Radiol* (1973) 46:148–9.

Andreasen NC, I don't believe in late onset schizophrenia. In: Howard R, Rabins PV, Castle DJ, eds, *Late Onset Schizophrenia* (Wrightson Biomedical Publishing: Petersfield: 1999).

Arndt S, Cohen G, Alliger RJ et al, Problems with ratio and proportion measures of imaged cerebral structures, *Psychiatry Res* (1991) 40:79–89.

Awad J, Spetzler R, Hodak J et al, Incidental lesions noted on magnetic resonance imaging of the brain: prevalence and clinical significance in various age groups, *Neurosurgery* (1987) 20:222–6.

Barak Y, Aizenberg D, Mirecki I et al, Very late-onset schizophrenia-like psychosis: clinical and imaging characteristics in comparison with elderly patients with schizophrenia, *J Nerv Ment Dis* (2002) 190:733–6.

Barta PE, Powers RE, Aylward EH et al, Quantitative MRI volume changes in late onset schizophrenia and Alzheimer's disease compared to normal controls, *Psychiatry Res* (1997) 68:65–75.

Bartzokis G, Schizophrenia: breakdown in the well-regulated lifelong process of brain development and maturation, *Neuropsychopharmacology* (2002) 27:672–83.

Berman KF, Doran AR, Pickar D, Weinberger DR, Is the mechanism of prefrontal hypofunction in depression the same as in schizophrenia? Regional cerebral blood flow during cognitive activation, *Br J Psychiatry* (1993) 162:183–92.

Berman KF, Torrey EF, Daniel DG, Weinberger DR, Regional cerebral blood flow in monozygotic twins discordant and concordant for schizophrenia, *Arch Gen Psychiatry* (1992) 49:927–34.

Bondareff W, Raval J, Woo B et al, Magnetic resonance imaging and the severity of dementia in older adults, *Arch Gen Psychiatry* (1990) 47:47–51.

Bornstein R, Schwartzkopf V, Olson S, Nasrallah H, Third ventricle enlargement and neuropsychological deficit in schizophrenia, *Biol Psychiatry* (1992) 31:954–61.

Bradley W, Waluch V, Brant-Zawadzki M et al, Patchy periventricular white matter lesions in the elderly: a common observation during NMR imaging, *Noninvasive Imaging* (1984) 1:35–41.

Braffman BH, Zimmerman RA, Trojanowski JQ, Brain MR: pathologic correlation with gross and histopathology. 1. Lacunar infarction and Virchow-Robin spaces, *Am J Roentgenol* (1988a) **151**:551–8.

Braffman B, Zimmerman R, Trojanowski J et al, Brain MR: pathologic correlation with gross and histopathology. 2. Hyperintense white matter foci in the elderly, *Am J Roentgenol* (1988b) **151**:559–66.

Breitner JC, Husain MM, Figiel GS et al, Cerebral white matter disease in late-onset paranoid psychosis, *Biol Psychiatry* (1990) **28**:266–74.

Burns A, Carrick J, Ames D et al, The cerebral cortical appearance in late paraphrenia, *Int J Geriatr Psychiatry* (1989) **4**:31–4.

Camargo EE, Brain SPECT in neurology and psychiatry, *J Nucl Med* (2001) **42**:611–23.

Casanova MF, Stevens JR, Brown R et al, Disentangling the pathology of schizophrenia and paraphrenia, *Acta Neuropathol* (2002) **103**:313–20.

Chance SA, Esiri MM, Crow TJ, Ventricular enlargement in schizophrenia: a primary change in the temporal lobe? *Schizophrenia Res* (2002) **62**:123–31.

Christiansen P, Larsson HB, Thomsen C et al, Age dependent white matter lesions and brain volume changes in healthy volunteers, *Acta Radiol* (1994) **35**:117–22.

Coffey CE, Figiel GS, Djahg WT, Weiner RD, Subcortical hyperintensity on magnetic resonance imaging: a comparison of normal and depressed elderly subjects, *Am J Psychiatry* (1990) **147**:187–9.

Corey-Bloom J, Jernigan T, Archibald S et al, Quantitative magnetic resonance imaging of the brain in late-life schizophrenia, *Am J Psychiatry* (1995) **152**:447–9.

Davis K, Stewart D, Friedman J et al, White matter changes in schizophrenia: evidence for myelin-related dysfunction, *Arch Gen Psychiatry* (2003) **60**:443–56.

Deicken RF, Johnson C, Pegues M, Proton magnetic resonance spectroscopy of the human brain in schizophrenia, *Rev Neurosci* (2000) **11**:147–58.

Deicken R, Reus V, Manfredi L, Wolkowitz O, MRI deep white matter intensity in a psychiatric population, *Biol Psychiatry* (1991) **29**:918–22.

Delamillieure P, Constans JM, Fernandez J et al, Proton magnetic resonance spectroscopy (1H MRS) in schizophrenia: investigation of the right and left hippocampus, thalamus, and prefrontal cortex, *Schizophrenia Bull* (2002) **28**:329–39.

Dennert J, Andreasen N, CT scanning and schizophrenia: a review, *Psychiatr Dev* (1983) **1**:105–22.

Dolan RJ, Calloway SP, Thacker PF, Mann AH, Cerebral cortical appearance in depressed subjects, *Psychol Med* (1986) **16**:775–9.

Fazekas F, Chawluck J, Alavi A et al, MR signal abnormalities at 1.5T in Alzheimer's dementia and normal ageing, *Am J Neuroradiol* (1987) **8**:421–6.

Fehr T, Kissler J, Moratti S et al, Source distribution of neuromagnetic slow waves and MEG-delta activity in schizophrenic patients, *Biol Psychiatry* (2001) **50**:108–16.

Firbank MJ, Minett T, O'Brien JT, Changes in DWI and MRS associated with white matter hyperintensities in elderly subjects, *Neurology* (2003) **61**:950–4.

Gaser C, Nenadic I, Buchsbaum BR et al, Ventricular enlargement in schizophrenia related to volume reduction of the thalamus, striatum, and superior temporal cortex, *Am J Psychiatry* (2004) **161**:154–6.

Grafton S, Sumi S, Stimac G et al, Comparison of postmortem magnetic resonance imaging and neuropathologic findings in the cerebral white matter, *Arch Neurol* (1991) **48**:293–8.

Grossman H, Harris G, Jacobson S, Folstein M, The normal elderly. In: Ames D, Chiu E, eds, *Neuroimaging and the Psychiatry of Late Life* (Cambridge University Press: Cambridge, 1997) 77–100.

Gurvits TV, Shenton ME, Hokama H et al, Magnetic resonance imaging study of hippocampal volume in chronic, combat-related posttraumatic stress disorder, *Biol Psychiatry* (1996) **40**:1091–9.

Haug J, Pneumoencephalographic studies in mental disease, *Acta Psychiatr Scand* (1965) **38**:S1–S104.

Hershey L, Modic M, Greenough P, Jaffe D, Magnetic resonance imaging in vascular dementia, *Neurology* (1987) **37**:29–36.

Howard R, Almeida O, Levy R et al, Quantitative magnetic resonance imaging volumetry distinguishes delusional disorder from late-onset schizophrenia, *Br J Psychiatry* (1994) **165**:474–80.

Howard R, Cox T, Almeida O et al, White matter signal hyperintensities in the brains of patients with late paraphrenia and the normal, community-living elderly, *Biol Psychiatry* (1995a) **38**:86–91.

Howard R, Förstl H, Naguib M et al, First-rank symptoms of Schneider in late paraphrenia, *Br J Psychiatry* (1992) **160**:108–9.

Howard R, Mellers J, Petty R et al, Magnetic resonance imaging volumetric measurements of the superior temporal gyrus, hippocampus, parahippocampal gyrus, frontal and temporal lobes in late paraphrenia, *Psychol Med* (1995b) **25**:495–503.

Howard R, Rabins PV, Seeman MV, Jeste DV, Late-onset schizophrenia and very-late-onset schizophrenia-like psychosis: an international consensus. The International Late-Onset Schizophrenia Group, *Am J Psychiatry* (2000) **157**:172–8.

Jacoby RJ, Levy R, Computed tomography in the elderly. 2. Senile dementia, *Br J Psychiatry* (1980) **136**:256–69.

Jani J, Prettyman R, Aslam M et al, A retrospective study of neuroradiological abnormalities detected on structural magnetic resonance imaging of the brain in elderly patients with cognitive impairment, *Int J Geriatr Psychiatry* (2000) **15**:1054–60.

Jessen F, Scheef L, Germeshausen L et al, Reduced hippocampal activation during encoding and recognition of words in schizophrenia patients, *Am J Psychiatry* (2003) **160**:1305–12.

Jezzard P, Song AW, Technical foundations and pitfalls of clinical fMRI, *Neuroimage* (1996) **4**:S63–S75.

Kapellar P, McLean MA, Griffin CM et al, Preliminary evidence for neuronal damage in cortical grey matter and normal appearing white matter in short duration relapsing-remitting multiple sclerosis: a quantitative MR spectroscopic imaging study, *J Neurol* (2001) **248**:131–8.

Keshavan M, Mulsant B, Sweet R et al, MRI changes in schizophrenia in late life: a preliminary controlled study, *Psychiatry Res* (1996) **60**:117–23.

Kim JJ, Mohamed S, Andreasen NC et al, Regional neural dysfunctions in chronic schizophrenia studied with positron emission tomography, *Am J Psychiatry* (2000) **157**:542–8.

Kindermann SS, Karimi A, Symonds L et al, Review of functional magnetic resonance imaging in schizophrenia, *Schizophr Res* (1997) **27**:143–56.

Krausz Y, Bonne O, Marciano R et al, Brain SPECT imaging of neuropsychiatric disorders, *Eur J Radiol* (1996) **21**:183–7.

Kumar A, Neuroimaging and geriatric psychiatry in the new millennium: the promise, the reality, and the need for more integrated approaches, *Am J Geriatr Psychiatry* (2002) **10**:1–4.

Kumari V, Gray JA, Honey GD et al, Procedural learning in schizophrenia: a functional magnetic resonance imaging investigation, *Schizophr Res* (2002) **57**:97–107.

Leary SM, Silver NC, Stevenson VL et al, Magnetization transfer of normal appearing white matter in primary/progressive multiple sclerosis, *Multiple Sclerosis* (1999) **5**:313–16.

Lesser IM, Jeste DV, Boone KB et al, Late-onset psychotic disorder, not otherwise specified: clinical and neuroimaging findings, *Biol Psychiatry* (1992) **31**:319–423.

Lesser IM, Miller BL, Swartz JR et al, Brain imaging in late-life schizophrenia and related psychoses, *Schizophr Bull* (1993) **19**:773–82.

Levin JM, Ross MH, Renshaw PF, Clinical applications of functional MRI in neuropsychiatry, *J Neuropsychiatry Clin Neurosci* (1995) **7**:511–22.

Lewis S, The secondary schizophrenias. In: Hirsch S, Weinberger D, eds, *Schizophrenia* (Blackwell Science: Oxford, 1995).

Liddle PF, Pantelis C, Brain imaging in schizophrenia. In: Hirsch S, Weinberger D, eds, *Schizophrenia*, 2nd edn (Blackwell Science: Oxford, 2003) 403–17.

Lloyd AJ, Ferrier IN, Barber R et al, Hippocampal volume change in depression: late- and early-onset illness compared, *Br J Psychiatry* (2004) **184**:488–95.

Lock T, Abou-Saleh M, Edwards R, Psychiatry and the new magnetic resonance era, *Br J Psychiatry* (1990) **9**:S38–S55.

McCarley RW, Wible CG, Frumin M et al, MRI anatomy of schizophrenia, *Biol Psychiatry* (1999) **45**:1099–119.

Malhi GS, Valenzuela M, Wen W, Sachdev P, Magnetic resonance spectroscopy and its applications in psychiatry, *Aust N Z J Psychiatry* (2002) **36**:31–43.

Mark LP, Ulmer JL, The next step: anatomy of the white matter, *Am J Neuroradiol* (2004) **25**:667–8.

Miller BL, Benson DF, Cummings JL, Neshkes R, Late-life paraphrenia: an organic delusional syndrome, *J Clin Psychiatry* (1986) **47**:204–7.

Miller BL, Lesser IM, Boone KB et al, Brain white-matter lesions and psychosis, *Br J Psychiatry* (1989) **155**:73–8.

Miller BL, Lesser IM, Boone KB et al, Brain lesions and cognitive function in late-life psychosis, *Br J Psychiatry* (1991) **158**:76–82.

Miller B, Lesser IM, Mena I et al, Regional cerebral blood flow in late-life-onset psychosis, *Neuropsychiatry Neuropsychol Behav Neurol* (1992) **5**:132–7.

Naguib M, Levy R, Late paraphrenia: neuropsychological impairment and structural brain abnormalities on computed tomography, *Int Geriatr Psychiatry* (1987) **2**:82–90.

Nelson MD, Saykin AJ, Flashman LA, Riordan HJ, Hippocampal volume reduction in schizophrenia as assessed by magnetic resonance imaging: a meta-analytic study, *Arch Gen Psychiatry* (1998) **55**:433–40.

O'Brien J, Desmond P, Ames D et al, A magnetic resonance imaging study of white matter lesions in depression and Alzheimer's disease, *Br J Psychiatry* (1996) **168**:477–85.

Palmer B, Heaton S, Jeste D, Older patients with schizophrenia: challenges in the coming decades, *Psychiatr Serv* (1999) **50**:1178–83.

Pantelis C, Velakoulis D, McGorry P et al, Neuroanatomical abnormalities before and after onset of psychosis: a cross-sectional and longitudinal MRI comparison, *Lancet* (2003a) **361**:281–8.

Pantelis C, Yucel M, Wood S et al, Early and late neurodevelopmental disturbances in schizophrenia and their functional consequences, *ANZJ Psych* (2003b) **37**:399–406.

Parsey R, Mann J, Applications of position emission tomography in psychiatry, *Semin Nucl Med* (2003) **33**:129–35.

Pearlson GD, Tune LE, Wong DF et al, Quantitative D2 dopamine receptor PET and structural MRI changes in late-onset schizophrenia, *Schizophr Bull* (1993) **19**:783–95.

Pilowsky LS, Costa DC, Ell PJ et al, D2 dopamine receptor binding in the basal ganglia of antipsychotic-free schizophrenic patients. An 123I-IBZM single photon emission computerised tomographic study, *Br J Psychiatry* (1994) **164**:16–26.

Rabins PV, Pearlson GD, Aylward E et al, Cortical magnetic resonance imaging changes in elderly inpatients with major depression, *Am J Psychiatry* (1991) **148**:617–20.

Rabins P, Pearlson G, Jayaram G et al, Increased ventricle-to-brain ratio in late-onset schizophrenia, *Am J Psychiatry* (1987) **144**:1216–18.

Rabins PV, Aylward E, Holroyd S, Pearlson G, MRI findings differentiate between late-onset schizophrenia and late-life mood disorder, *Int J Geriatr Psychiatry* (2000) 15:954–60.

Reite M, Teale P, Rojas DC, Magnetoencephalography: applications in psychiatry, *Biol Psychiatry* (1999) **45**:1553–63.

Reite M, Teale P, Sheeder J et al, Neuropsychiatric applications of MEG, *Electroencephalogr Clin Neurophysiol* (1996) **S47**:363–82.

Riecher-Rössler A, Häfner H, Häfner-Ranabauer W et al, Late-onset schizophrenia versus paranoid psychoses: a valid diagnostic distinction?, *Am J Geriatr Psychiatry* (2003) **11**:595–604.

Rivkin P, Kraut M, Barta P et al, White matter hyperintensity volume in late-onset and early-onset schizophrenia, *Int J Geriatr Psychiatry* (2000) 15:1085–9.

Sachdev P, Brodaty H, Mid-sagittal anatomy in late-onset schizophrenia, *Psychol Med* (1999a) **29**:963–70.

Sachdev P, Brodaty H, Quantitative study of signal hyperintensities on T2-weighted magnetic resonance imaging in late-onset schizophrenia, *Am J Psychiatry* (1999b) **156**:1958–67.

Sachdev P, Brodaty H, Rose N, Cathcart S, Schizophrenia with onset after age 50 years. 2: Neurological, neuropsychological and MRI investigation, *Br J Psychiatry* (1999a) **175**:416–21.

Sachdev P, Brodaty H, Rose N, Haindl W, Regional cerebral blood flow in late-onset schizophrenia: a SPECT study using 99mTc-HMPAO, *Schizophr Res* (1997) 27:105–17.

Sachdev P, Cathcart S, Shnier R et al, Reliability and validity of ratings of signal hyperintensities on MRi by visual inspection and computerised measurement, *Psychiatry Res* (1999b) 92:103–15.

Sack AT, Linden DE, Combining transcranial magnetic stimulation and functional imaging in cognitive brain research: possibilities and limitations, *Brain Res Rev* (2003) **43**:41–56.

Shelton RC, Weinberger DR, X-ray computerized tomography studies in schizophrenia: a review and synthesis. In: Nasrallah HA, Weinberger DR, eds, *Handbook of Schizophrenia: The Neuropathology of Schizophrenia* (Elsevier Science: New York, 1986) 207–25.

Shenton ME, Dickey CC, Frumin M, McCarley RW, A review of MRI findings in schizophrenia, *Schizophr Res* (2001) **49**:1–52.

Shoghi-Jadid K, Small GW, Agdeppa ED et al, Localization of neurofibrillary tangles and beta-amyloid plaques in the brains of living patients with alzheimer disease, *Am J Geriatr Psychiatry* (2002) **10**:24–35.

Soares JC, Innis RB, Neurochemical brain imaging investigations of schizophrenia, *Biol Psychiatry* (1999) **46**:600–15.

Swayze V, Andreasen N, Alliger R et al, Structural brain abnormalities in bipolar affective disorder, *Arch Gen Psychiatry* (1990) **47**:1054–9.

Symonds LL, Olichney JM, Jernigan TL et al, Lack of clinically significant gross structural abnormalities in MRIs of older patients with schizophrenia and related psychoses, *J Neuropsychiatry Clin Neurosci* (1997) 9:251–8.

Taylor W, Hsu E, Krishnan K, MacFall J, Diffusion tensor imaging: background, potential, and utility in psychiatric research, *Biol Psychiatry* (2004) **55**:201–7.

Thomas A, O'Brien J, Barber R et al, A neuropathological study of periventricular white matter hyperintensities in major depression, *J Affect Disord* (2003) 76:49–54.

Tonkonogy JM, Geller JL, Late-onset paranoid psychosis as a distinct clinicopathologic entity: magnetic resonance imaging data in elderly patients with paranoid psychosis of late onset and schizophrenia of early onset, *Neuropsychiatry, Neuropsychol Behav Neurol* (1999) 12:230–5.

Trimble M, First-rank symptoms of Schneider: a new perspective?, *Br J Psychiatry* (1990) **156**:195–200.

Vance AL, Velakoulis D, Maruff P et al, Magnetic resonance spectroscopy and schizophrenia: what have we learnt?, *Aust N Z J Psychiatry* (2000) **34**:14–25.

Vasile R, Single photon emission computed tomography in psychiatry: current perspectives, *Harvard Rev Psychiatry* (1996) **4**:27–38.

Velakoulis D, Pantelis C, McGorry PD et al, Hippocampal volume in first-episode psychoses and chronic schizophrenia: a high-resolution magnetic resonance imaging study, *Arch Gen Psychiatry* (1999) **56**:133–41.

Velakoulis D, Wood S, McGorry P, Pantelis C, Evidence for progression of brain structural abnormalities in schizophrenia: beyond the neurodevelopmental model, *Aust N Z J Psychiatry* (2000) **34** (suppl):S113–S126.

Velakoulis D, Wood S, Smith D et al, Increased duration of illness is associated with reduced volume in right medial temporal/anterior cingulate grey matter in patients with chronic schizophrenia, *Schizophr Res* (2002) **57**:43–9.

Walter H, Wunderlich AP, Blankenhorn M et al, No hypofrontality, but absence of prefrontal lateralization comparing verbal and spatial working memory in schizophrenia, *Schizophr Res* (2003) **61**:175–84.

Ward KE, Friedman L, Wise A, Schulz SC, Meta-analysis of brain and cranial size in schizophrenia, *Schizophr Res* (1996) **22**:197–213.

Weinberger DR, Torrey EF, Neophytides AN, Wyatt RJ, Structural abnormalities in the cerebral cortex of chronic schizophrenic patients, *Arch Gen Psychiatry* (1979) **36**:935–9.

Wen W, Sachdev P, The topography of white matter hyperintensities on brain MRI in healthy 60- to 64-year-old individuals, *Neuroimage* (2004) **22**:144–54.

Whittal KP, MacKay AL, Li DK et al, Normal appearing white matter in multiple sclerosis has heterogeneous, diffusely prolonged T2, *Magn Reson Med* (2002) **47**:403–8.

Wishart HA, Saykin AJ, McAllister TW, Functional magnetic resonance imaging: emerging clinical applications, *Curr Psychiatry Reports* (2002) **4**:338–45.

Woods BT, Douglass A, Gescuk B, Is the VBR still a useful measure of changes in the cerebral ventricles?, *Psychiatry Res* (1991) **40**:1–10.

chapter 5

The neuropsychology of late-onset schizophrenia

Osvaldo P. Almeida

The first systematic description of paranoid features with onset in later life was published by Kleist in 1913 under the title of *Involutional Paranoia*. He speculated on the possible contribution of organic factors to the development of psychotic symptoms and concluded that involutional paranoia was unlikely to be caused by primary degenerative or progressive cerebrovascular disease. In 1952, Roth and Morrisey described a group of 12 elderly patients with a well-organized system of paranoid delusions in whom signs of 'senility' were absent (Roth and Morrisey, 1952). The authors emphasized that the disorder developed in the setting of preserved intellect (i.e. cognitive function). Subsequently, Roth (1955) showed that these patients followed a course that was different from that experienced by people with dementia and affective illness with regard to mortality and symptomatological remission after a follow-up period of two years. Kay and Roth (1961) later introduced the concept of 'late paraphrenia' as a 'suitable descriptive term, without prejudice as to etiology, for all cases with a paranoid symptom-complex in which signs of organic dementia or sustained confusion were absent, and in which the condition was judged from the content of the delusional and hallucinatory symptoms not to be due to a primary affective disorder'. However, since its inception, the concept of late paraphrenia was surrounded by controversy, as many considered the disorder to be nothing but the expression of schizophrenia in later life (e.g. Fish, 1960).

This brief historical introduction highlights two of the key issues involving the concept of late-onset schizophrenia-spectrum disorders (LOS): (1) the relationship with early-onset schizophrenia (EOS) and, (2) the relationship with neurodegenerative conditions. This chapter aims to review the neuropsychological features of LOS, compare them with the neuropsychological profile of people with EOS, and clarify whether currently available evidence indicates that LOS is associated with progressive cognitive decline.

The neuropsychology of LOS

The first systematic assessment of individuals with LOS was published in 1953 by Hopkins and Roth. They used the vocabulary subtest from the Wechsler-Bellevue Scale, a short form of the Raven's Progressive Matrices, and a general test for the assessment of orientation and information to evaluate the cognitive performance of 12 subjects with LOS. Their performance was similar to that of older adults with depression, but better than those with 'senile' or 'vascular' dementia in all three tests. Thirty-four years later, Naguib and Levy (1987) compared the cognitive performance of 43 patients with that of healthy controls and concluded that LOS was associated with impoverished performance on relatively simple tests such as the Mental Test Score and Digit Copying Test.

In the early 1990s Miller et al (1991) published a detailed neuropsychological investigation of patients with LOS (mean age 60.1 years), which included the Mini-mental State Examination (MMSE), Wechsler Adult Intelligence Scale-Revised, Wisconsin Card Sorting Test, Logical Memory and Visual Reproduction from the Wechsler Memory Scale, verbal fluency, the Stroop Test and the Warrington Recognition Memory Test. Patients performed worse than their age-matched controls in all tasks, although the analyses were not adjusted for education or premorbid intelligence. Further investigations of the cognitive deficits associated with LOS confirmed that, compared with age-, gender-, education- and premorbid intelligence-matched controls, older people with LOS display a pattern of generalized cognitive impairment (Sachdev et al, 1999), although the deficits seem to be qualitatively different from those observed among patients with dementia. For example, Almeida et al (1995a) found that their 40 patients with LOS performed significantly worse than 33 controls on the Cambridge Cognitive Examination for the Elderly (CAMCOG – a measure of general cognitive ability), the Recognition Memory Test, verbal fluency, and on computerized measures of planning, working memory, and delayed recall. However, contrary to what had been described for older people with Alzheimer's disease (AD), patients' deficits in delayed recall were not time-dependent (i.e. deficits did not increase proportionally more for patients than for controls with increasing delay of recall).

To date, few studies have directly compared the neuropsychological performance of older adults with schizophrenia and AD (none involving LOS). McBride et al (2002) confirmed that their 44 institutionalized elderly patients with chronic schizophrenia showed a pattern of generalized cognitive impairment that involved memory, language, verbal fluency, and constructional skills. However, they observed that, compared with 43 patients with AD matched for age, gender, education, ethnic origin and total MMSE score, patients with schizophrenia had significantly better performance on tests involving delayed recall, but worse performance on naming. Overall, the results of this study showed that chronic schizophrenia is associated with marked cognitive impairment, but the profile of neuropsychological deficits among these patients is different from that observed among people with AD.

In summary, LOS is associated with a pattern of generalized cognitive impairment that involves memory, visuospatial abilities, psychomotor speed, and executive functions. Although the cognitive deficits of schizophrenia are not typical of 'dementia', their consequences are of great clinical relevance. Evans et al (2003) found that the functional capacity of 93 patients with schizophrenia or schizoaffective disorder (mean age = 57.2 ± 9.1 years) is directly correlated with their cognitive performance, which confirmed the findings of previous studies indicating that functional impairment in schizophrenia is very closely related to the severity of the cognitive deficits (Kurtz et al, 2001).

Comparing the neuropsychological deficits of schizophrenia with early and late onset

Early-onset schizophrenia is associated with a pervasive pattern of generalized cognitive impairment that includes deficits in memory, attention, set-shifting, language, visuospatial abilities, psychomotor speed, and planning (Heinrichs and Zakzanis, 1998). Recently published findings from studies investigating the neuropsychological profile of young people with first-episode schizophrenia indicate that this pattern of generalized cognitive impairment is already present at the time of illness onset. For example, Bilder et al (2000) reported a detailed neuropsychological evaluation of 94 patients with first-episode schizophrenia (mean age = 25.7 ± 6.3 years) and 36 age- and gender-matched healthy controls. Forty-one tests were used to assess language, memory, attention, executive function, motor and visuospatial skills, as well as general cognitive ability (IQ and MMSE). Patients had significantly lower scores than controls in all individual tasks. In fact, the scores of patients with first-episode schizophrenia on language, memory, attention, executive function, motor and visuospatial skills were on average 1.2–1.8 standard deviations lower than the scores of controls.

In many respects, the cognitive profile of subjects with EOS and LOS is similar, although direct between-group comparison has been almost unavailable. This issue was partly addressed by Sachdev et al (1999). They found that the cognitive performance of their 27 subjects with LOS was in all respects comparable to that of 30 subjects with EOS on tests assessing speed of information processing, memory, and executive function. Of note, the neuropsychological scores of both patient groups were significantly worse than the results obtained by 34 healthy controls.

In summary, subjects with EOS and LOS display a pattern of generalized cognitive impairment that seems to be qualitatively and quantitatively similar, although currently available evidence is mostly indirect rather than originating from the direct comparison between these two patient groups.

LOS, cognitive decline and dementia

LOS and cognitive decline

When Kraepelin first introduced the concept of *dementia praecox* (now known as schizophrenia), he highlighted two essential core features of the condition: functional and intellectual decline. As previously described, both EOS and LOS are associated with a pattern of generalized cognitive impairment which, as we have discussed in a separate publication, represents a decline from a relatively normal previous level of function (Almeida and Howard, 2005). A related and equally important question that researchers have been trying to answer for over a century now is whether schizophrenia leads to cognitive decline and, ultimately, dementia.

Hoff et al (1999) prospectively monitored the cognitive abilities of 42 patients with first-episode EOS and 16 healthy controls. They reported that the scores of patients for tasks assessing language, verbal and spatial memory, executive function, psychomotor speed, and sensory perception remained relatively stable at 1–1.5 standard deviations below the baseline level of performance of controls during the follow-up period of 5 years. Other studies have confirmed that the cognitive abilities of patients with first-episode schizophrenia do not deteriorate over time – on the contrary, they may actually improve with treatment (Gold et al, 1999).

The first prospective follow-up study of subjects with LOS was reported by Hymas et al in 1989. Thirty-one subjects from the original sample of 43 patients originally examined by Naguib and Levy (1987) were still alive after a follow-up period of 3.7 years – 45% showed significant cognitive deterioration on the Mental Test Score, although only 6% of them scored below the cut-off point for dementia. Unfortunately, the interpretation of these results is hampered by the fact that a staggering 26% of patients from the original sample had died prior to the second assessment. More recently, Palmer et al (2003) followed up for two years a group of 37 outpatients with LOS (defined as schizophrenia-spectrum disorder starting after the age of 45), 69 patients with EOS and 67 individuals with AD. They found that subjects with LOS or EOS and controls experienced very limited changes in cognitive function over two years, which compared favorably with the obvious cognitive decline observed among older adults with AD. The authors concluded that LOS is a static encepalopathy, not a neurodegenerative disorder.

In contrast, Brodaty et al (2003) reported that their 19 patients with LOS (defined as schizophrenia starting after the age of 50) showed greater deterioration than controls on the MMSE score over five years. However, patients recruited into this study had had significantly less years of education and lower baseline MMSE scores than controls (mean MMSE = 25.5 ± 3.5 vs 29.7 ± 1.0), which is likely to have biased the overall results of the study in favor of the control group.

In summary, currently available evidence suggests that the cognitive deficits of EOS are not progressive in nature, whereas the long-term cognitive outcome of older adults with LOS remains unclear.

Schizophrenia and dementia

Preliminary evidence suggests that the risk of functional decline among people with schizophrenia increases with increasing age after the age of 70. Friedman et al (2001) monitored the functional decline of 107 patients with schizophrenia aged 20–80 over a six-year period. They reported that at around the age of 80, subjects with schizophrenia reached the same level of functional impairment observed among patients with AD. The authors concluded that the cognitive and functional status of institutionalized patients with schizophrenia is very stable until very late in life, when a rapid decline in functional capacity becomes apparent.

A recently published chart review of the long-term outcome of 48 subjects with LOS (mean age at onset = 69.4, age at initial contact = 73.3) and

48 patients with a major depressive disorder (age = 73.2) showed that more than 50% of patients with LOS had met DSM-IV diagnostic criteria for dementia 10 years after the initial contact with the service (Rabins and Lavrisha, 2003). There is also observational evidence that delusions and hallucinations are associated with increased risk of incident dementia among community-dwelling people aged 85 or over (Östling and Skoog, 2002), suggesting that, as is the case for depression (Jorm, 2001), in some people, LOS may represent a prodrome of dementia.

However, the results of neuropathological investigations of people with schizophrenia available to date have failed to demonstrate the presence of significant AD-related pathology. For example, Purohit et al (1998) did not find an excessive number of senile plaques and neurofibrillary tangles, or neuronal loss in the brains of 100 patients with schizophrenia aged 52–101 at the time of death. Likewise, Arnold et al (1998) found that their 23 elderly patients with schizophrenia had no more neurodegenerative lesions than 14 nondemented controls. More recently, Religa et al (2003) reported that the brain concentration of β-amyloid 40 and β-amyloid 42 was significantly lower among patients with schizophrenia and controls than among subjects with AD (β-amyloid is thought to be a key component of the pathogenetic process that ultimately leads to the development of AD). Taken together, these results show that schizophrenia is not associated with increased neurodegeneration, but do not clarify whether such findings can be extended to older adults with late onset of illness.

Two neuropathological investigations of subjects with LOS threw some light on this issue. The first was published in the late 1960s by Blessed et al (1968). They examined the brains of five people with LOS and found that the number of senile plaques in their cerebral cortex was much lower than in patients with dementia, but not significantly different from the number of plaques found among older adults with depression and controls. In a more recent study, Casanova et al (2002) reported that the brains of their 64 patients with schizophrenia showed significantly more tau pathology than the brains of controls, although the severity of these changes did not reach the threshold for the neuropathological diagnosis of AD (tau is a microtubule-associated protein that plays a critical role in the formation of neurofibrillary tangles). The authors further reported that amyloid deposits were sparse or absent in this group of patients and that there were no obvious neuropathological differences between the brains of patients with EOS andf LOS (defined as onset of illness at or after the age of 40). Casanova et al (2002) concluded that schizophrenia is associated with mild neuronal cytoskeletal disruption of limbic areas.

In summary, currently available neuropathological findings are consistent with the hypothesis that schizophrenia is not a progressive neurodegenerative condition. However, most studies reported to date have limited their investigation to the brains of older adults with a long-standing history of schizophrenia, not to people with LOS. In addition, the only two studies that systematically described the neuropathological findings associated with LOS have used different definitions of LOS. Nonetheless, their results seem to confirm that LOS is not associated with senile plaques or obvious amyloid pathology, which suggests that the neuropathological processes underlying the expression of LOS and AD are not the same.

Conclusion

Delusions and hallucinations are not uncommon among older adults. Their emergence in later life, however, lacks diagnostic specificity and may be the symptomatological expression of a mood disorder, AD, dementia with Lewy bodies, vascular dementia, fronto-temporal dementia, delirium, drug use and schizophrenia-spectrum disorders, among others. Therefore, misclassification is likely to occur, particularly when psychotic symptoms arise during or after the eighth decade of life. If such a premise is true, then the neuropsychological evaluation of people with LOS will reflect the heterogeneity of this population, as previously suggested (Almeida et al, 1995b). Consequently, subjects with LOS may experience a significantly higher rate of cognitive decline and a disproportionately high rate of conversion to dementia over time (e.g. Östling and Skoog, 2002).

Investigations using a relatively young age at onset to define LOS (40 or 45 years) are less likely to be susceptible to this type of recruitment bias. The results of such studies consistently show that there is nothing special about the neuropsychological profile of LOS: (1) LOS and EOS display the same pattern of generalized cognitive impairment, (2) there is no evidence of a disproportionately higher rate of cognitive decline over time in the two patient groups and, (3) there is no excess of dementia cases among patients with EOS or LOS with increasing age.

References

Almeida OP, Howard R, Schizophrenia, cognitive impairment and dementia. In: O'Brien JT, Ames D, Burns A, eds, *Dementia*, 3rd edn (Hodder: London, 2005).

Almeida OP, Howard R, Levy R et al, Cognitive features of psychotic states arising in late life (late paraphrenia), *Psychol Med* (1995a) 25:685–98.

Almeida OP, Howard R, Levy R et al, Clinical and cognitive diversity of psychotic states arising in late life (late paraphrenia), *Psychol Med* (1995b) 25:699–714.

Arnold SE, Trojanowski JQ, Gur RE et al, Absence of neurodegeneration and neural injury in the cerebral cortex in a sample of elderly patients with schizophrenia, *Arch Gen Psychiatry* (1998) 55:225–32.

Bilder RM, Goldman RS, Robinson D et al, Neuropsychology of first-episode schizophrenia: initial characterization and clinical correlates, *Am J Psychiatry* (2000) 157:549–59.

Blessed G, Tomlinson BE, Roth M, The association between quantitative measures of dementia and of senile change in the cerebral grey matter of elderly subjects, *Br J Psychiatry* (1968) 114:797–811.

Brodaty H, Sachdev P, Kschera A et al, Long-term outcome of late-onset schizophrenia: 5-year follow-up study, *Br J Psychiatry* (2003) 183:212–19.

Casanova MF, Stevens JR, Brown R et al, Disentangling the pathology of schizophrenia and paraphrenia, *Acta Neuropathol* (2002) 103:313–20.

Evans JD, Heaton RK, Paulsen JS et al, The relationship of neuropsychological abilities to specific domains of functional capacity in older schizophrenia patients, *Biol Psychiatry* (2003) 53:422–30.

Fish F, Senile schizophrenia, *J Ment Sci* (1960) 106:938–46.

Friedman JI, Harvey PD, Coleman T et al, Six-year follow-up study of cognitive and functional status across the lifespan in schizophrenia: a comparison with Alzheimer's disease and normal aging, *Am J Psychiatry* (2001) 158:1441–8.

Gold S, Arndt S, Nopoulos P et al, Longitudinal study of cognitive function in first-episode and recent-onset schizophrenia, *Am J Psychiatry* (1999) 156:1342–8.

Heinrichs RW, Zakzanis KK, Neurocognitive deficit in schizophrenia: a quantitative review of the evidence, *Neuropsychology* (1998) 12:426–45.

Hoff AL, Sakuma M, Wieneke M et al, Longitudinal neuropsychological follow-up study of patients with first-episode schizophrenia, *Am J Psychiatry* (1999) 156:1336–41.

Hopkins B, Roth M, Psychological test performance in patients over sixty. II. Paraphrenia, arteriosclerotic psychosis and acute confusion, *J Ment Sci* (1953) 99:451–63.

Hymas N, Naguib M, Levy R, Late paraphrenia: a follow-up study, *Int J Geriatr Psychiatry* (1989) 4:23–9.

Jorm AF, History of depression as a risk factor for dementia: an updated review, *Aust N Z J Psychiatry* (2001) 35:776–81.

Kay DWK, Roth M, Environmental and hereditary factors in the schizophrenias of old age ('late paraphrenia') and their bearing on the general problem of causation in schizophrenia, *J Ment Sci* (1961) 107:649–86.

Kleist K, Is involutional paranoia due to an organic-destructive brain process. *Die involutionsparanoia Allgemeine, Zeitschrift für Psychiatrie* (translated by Förstl H, Howard R, Ameida OP, et al). In: Katona C, Levy R, eds, *Delusions and Hallucinations in Old Age* (Gaskell: London, 1992) 165–6.

Kurtz MM, Moberg PJ, Mozely LH et al, Cognitive impairment and functional status in elderly institutionalized patients with schizophrenia, *Int J Geriatr Psychiatry* (2001) 16:631–8.

McBride T, Moberg PJ, Arnold SE et al, Neuropsychological functioning in elderly patients with schizophrenia and Alzheimer's disease, *Schizophr Res* (2002) 55:217–27.

Miller BL, Lesser IM, Boone KB et al, Brain lesions and cognitive function in late-life psychosis, *Br J Psychiatry* (1991) 158:76–82.

Naguib M, Levy R, Late paraphrenia: neuropsychological impairment and structural brain abnormalities on computed tomography, *Int J Geriatr Psychiatry* (1987) 2:83–90.

Östling S, Skoog I, Psychotic symptoms and paranoid ideation in a nondemented population-based sample of the very old, *Arch Gen Psychiatry* (2002) 59:53–9.

Palmer BW, Bondi MW, Twamley EW et al, Are late-onset schizophrenia spectrum disorders neurodegenerative conditions? Annual rates of change on two dementia measures, *J Neuropsychiatry Clin Neurosci* (2003) 15:45–52.

Purohit DP, Perl DP, Haroutunian V et al, Alzheimer disease and related neuro-degenerative diseases in elderly patients with schizophrenia: a post-mortem neuropathologic study of 100 cases, *Arch Gen Psychiatry* (1998) 55:205–11.

Rabins PV, Lavrisha M, Long-term follow-up and phenomenologic differences distinguish among late-onset schizophrenia, late-life depression and progressive dementia, *Am J Geriatr Psychiatry* (2003) 11:589–94.

Religa D, Laudon H, Styczynska M et al, Amyloid β pathology in Alzheimer's disease and schizophrenia, *Am J Psychiatry* (2003) 160:867–72.

Roth M, The natural history of mental disorders in old age, *J Ment Sci* (1955) 101:281–301.

Roth M, Morrisey J, Problems in the diagnosis and classification of mental disorders in old age, *J Ment Sci* (1952) 98:66–80.

Sachdev P, Broday H, Rose N, Cathcart S, Schizophrenia with onset after age 50 years. 2: Neurological, neuropsychological and MRI investigation, *Br J Psychiatry* (1999) 175:416–21.

Part II

Management of early- and late-onset schizophrenia

chapter 6

The use of antipsychotic medication for schizophrenia occurring in late life

Craig W. Ritchie

Introduction

With the exception of the common dementias, the range and type of psychiatric illness observed in the elderly is similar to that of younger populations. However, there are valid reasons why the etiology, prognosis, and treatment of conditions either persisting into late life or arising for the first time in the elderly are different from those noted in younger patients. This would argue for specific research into the therapies used in late-life mental illness, but sadly this evidence base is lacking. For the most part, our prescribing of neuroleptic medication to the elderly psychotic patient is based on the conclusions from studies in younger populations. This is particularly frustrating given that the perceived benefits of newer antipsychotics (management of negative and cognitive symptoms and reduced risk of motor side effects) would be especially relevant to an elderly population.

This chapter will discuss the reasons for the limited evidence base, before summarizing the reasons why specific studies are merited in an elderly population of people with schizophrenia. It will then review the current available literature and in doing so highlight the continuing gaps in our knowledge. Finally, the management of schizophrenia in the elderly population will be discussed.

Why the lack of evidence?

It is not a licensing requirement for a new antipsychotic drug that it be tested specifically in the elderly either for its initial licensing or indeed for its later use in the elderly. For this reason almost all of the pivotal licensing trials for the new antipsychotics have actively excluded patients 65 years old and older. From a commercial perspective, the potential efficacy and safety differences between younger and older patients preclude including the elderly in these licensing studies. Including elderly patients would increase the heterogeneity of the trial sample at baseline, which would reduce the power to detect differences between any new drug and a placebo or active comparator. A much larger sample would be required to show efficacy, which would be more costly and commercially unnecessary.

It is disappointing, however, that this heterogeneity is not then addressed by subsequent large, well-designed Phase IV studies. Only two double-blind, randomized controlled trials in the elderly population with schizophrenia have been published – comparing olanzapine with risperidone (Jeste et al, 2003) and comparing olanzapine with haloperidol (Kennedy et al, 2003). Both were particularly short trials, which limited their scope considerably.

Differences between the old and young – why should there be a specific evidence base?

It is likely that general conclusions from studies in younger populations with schizophrenia will be reasonably valid in the elderly as there are more similarities than differences between the two groups. However, to optimize treatments in terms of both efficacy and minimization of risk, four things must be considered:

1. different clinical picture
2. different etiology of illness
3. different type and frequency of concomitant medical problems
4. different pharmacokinetic and pharmacodynamic profiles.

Points 1–3 will be dealt with in detail later in the chapter.

Pharmacokinetic and pharmacodynamic considerations in managing schizophrenia in the elderly

In general, smaller doses of psychotropic drugs are required in the elderly to achieve the same plasma levels observed in younger populations. Although Phase 1 data are seldom published, it is unlikely that during Phase 1 testing of new compounds for schizophrenia specific trials are undertaken in the elderly. Consideration of what constitutes the optimal dose must then take into account general considerations regarding pharmacokinetic changes which result from aging. Occasionally, Phase IV studies are available which will guide prescribing.

Invariably antipsychotic drugs are given orally or by intramuscular injection. Absorption of drugs orally is rarely affected by aging, although as intramuscular absorption from muscle tissue is affected by blood flow, a reduction in blood flow to the site of injection could in theory reduce the rate of drug absorption and hence prolong the activity of the depot.

As all psychotropic drugs are highly lipophilic, they are readily distributed into body fat. In general, aging is associated with a reduction in the proportion of an individual's body fat, which would mean that there would be greater bioavailability of the same dose of drug in an older compared with a younger person. In reality though, distribution into body fat tends to have little effect on the availability of drug due to the relatively poor blood supply of fat.

The most important consideration affecting dosing in the elderly is metabolism and excretion. Almost all psychotropic drugs and all neuroleptics undergo Phase 1 oxidative reactions in the liver. This reaction involves various components of the cytochrome P450 system, which can become less effective as one ages. However, decline in the function of this system is not predictable and there is great inter-individual variation in the function of this metabolic process. Moreover this system is affected by other psychotropic and nonpsychotropic drugs, which may influence the metabolism of antipsychotics. Phase 1 studies are often conducted in populations with hepatic impairment and it is clear from these that a reduction in dose of neuroleptics medication is necessary where impairment is present. However, liver function tests are a poor guide to the viability of the cytochrome P450 system and clinicians should not derive comfort that the system is working well on the basis of normal liver function tests.

Most neuroleptics then undergo polarization through Phase 2 reactions, e.g. glucuronation, which again take place predominantly in the liver.

Abnormalities in liver function tests are more closely associated with impairment in this enzymic activity. As the products of Phase 1 reactions are often still active, a failing in Phase 2 metabolism could lead to an accumulation of active metabolites. Once polarized (and inactivated) by Phase 2 reactions, the drug is then excreted by the kidney.

Renal excretion accounts for the vast majority of the clearance of neuroleptics drugs from the body, as very few of these drugs undergo biliary secretion and therefore excretion in feces.

A further consideration is that the elderly are more likely than younger populations to be on other medications, both psychotropic and nonpsychotropic. There is therefore a greater risk of drug–drug interactions taking place. Finally, pharmacodynamic considerations have to be acknowledged. The pharmacodynamics of a drug is 'what the drug does to the body'. Invariably in psychiatry this means what a drug does to the neuron and/or its products as a result of binding to neuroreceptors.

As a consequence of the normal neurodegeneration associated with aging there tends to be an associated decrease in the number of any given neuroreceptors. As a consequence the same dose of drug as used in a younger population will occupy a greater proportion of receptors leading to a greater effect.

This diminution of receptor number and altered pharmacokinetic profile in the elderly underpins the increased sensitivity that the elderly have in developing side effects such as parkinsonism with dopamine blockade in the substantia nigra and confusion with nicotinic blockade in cortical neurons.

Different clinical picture
Schizophrenia in late life is of two broad types:

- that which has developed or emerged for the first time in late life (often referred to as late paraphrenia)
- that which has persisted from onset as a young adult, through the patient's adult years into late life.

The clinical picture of these two groups is quite different.

It is beyond the scope of this particular chapter to discuss in detail these differences; for a review see Roth and Kay (1998) and Chapters 1 and 2 of this book. Table 6.1 highlights the key differences and similarities between the two populations. This can then be contrasted with the picture presented in younger patients with schizophrenia.

Table 6.1 Comparisons between late-onset, persistent, and early-onset schizophrenia

Parameter	Late-onset	Persistent disease into late life	Schizophrenia in general adult population (EOS)
Clinical features			
Positive Symptoms	+++	+	++
Negative Symptoms	+/−	++	+
Thought Disorder	−	++	+
Affective Symptoms	+	+	+
Cognitive Symptoms	++	+++	+
Diagnostic subtype	Paranoid/ delusional disorder	Residual	Paranoid
Proposed etiology	Neurodegenerative	Neurodevelopmental plus secondary neurodegenerative	Neurodevelopmental
Prognosis and response to drug treatment	Stable non-progressive with reasonably high function. Limited response to drug treatment	Nonprogressive, although with high level of disability. Good response to atypical drugs	Variable. One-third of patients progress to chronic illness. Prognosis improved with drug treatment

Different etiology

Most authors agree that the etiology of schizophrenia is multifactorial involving both genetic and environmental components. In this regard the genetic vulnerability and environmental insults that impact upon any individual from gestation forward have led to the conclusion that early-onset schizophrenia is the result of neurodevelopmental problems triggered by environmental factors (Weinberger, 1987; Bullmore, et al, 1997). However, schizophrenia that develops in late life is less easily characterized as being due to neurodevelopmental abnormalities. There may well be a lifelong vulnerability to developing schizophrenia, although this etiological burden is not as heavy in elderly cases as it is in younger patients. There is then a trigger in later life for the development of a schizophrenic illness; this trigger could be organic in nature (Miller et al, 1991; Burns and Förstl, 1997). If, as is probably the case, schizophrenia of late life has a different etiology (possibly neurodegenerative) to younger-onset illness (neurodevelopmental), then it is clear that there may be different responses to pharmaceutical intervention.

Different type and frequency of concomitant medical problems

A final factor arguing for more specific investigation into the efficacy and safety of drug treatments in late-onset schizophrenia is the physical health of the elderly compared with younger populations. Despite the well-known associations between schizophrenia and poor physical health (Brown, 1997), it is clear that the elderly in any given population are more likely to have poorer physical health and be prescribed other psychotropic and nonpsychotropic medications.

There is then a strong need to understand the use of antipsychotic drugs in the presence of polypharmacy and renal, hepatic, and cognitive impairment. The most effective way to understand this is to undertake large critical evaluations of the safety of these drugs in this population.

What evidence does exist in the elderly?

Atypical antipsychotics are the predominant drug of choice in treating psychosis at all ages. Systematic reviews of their use in adult populations have shown them to be of proven efficacy in managing core symptoms of schizophrenia while having a significant benefit over conventional neuroleptics in terms of motor side effects (Geddes et al, 2000). This latter property should theoretically have particular application in the elderly who are as a group more susceptible to developing both parkinsonism (Sweet and Pollock, 1995) and dyskinetic movements (Jeste et al, 1995, 1999) than younger people with schizophrenia.

Clinical trials examining the use of olanzapine or risperidone in late-life schizophrenia tend to support this theory. However, these studies are imperfect for several reasons including: heterogeneous study population (Madhusoodanan et al, 1995, 2000; Joshi and Joshi, 1996; Davidson et al, 2000), retrospective design (Kiraly et al, 1998; Madhusoodanan et al, 1999a; Solomons and Geiger, 2000), single arm (Madhusoodanan et al, 1995, 1999b, 2000; Berman et al, 1996; Davidson et al, 2000; Solomons and Geiger, 2000), small sample size (Berman et al, 1996; 2000; Barak et al, 2002; Madhusoodanan et al, 1995; 2000), nonspecific or limited outcome measures (Kiraly et al, 1998), and short follow-up period (Madhusoodanan et al, 1999b; Jeste et al, 2003; Kennedy et al, 2003). Despite these limitations they have consistently indicated efficacy in improving core schizophrenic symptoms, reducing extra-pyramidal side effects (EPSE) and being well tolerated. More recent studies have compared olanzapine with haloperidol in both open label (Barak et al, 2002) and double-blind conditions (Kennedy et al, 2003) with both studies reporting superior efficacy and a reduction in motor side effects. Jeste et al (2003) reported on a large, multicenter study comparing olanzapine with risperidone over eight weeks under double-blind conditions. This study demonstrated reduction in both symptoms and side effects, although it did not demonstrate any significant within-group differences.

Our own work in a randomized, open-label study (Ritchie et al, 2003) suggested that both olanzapine and risperidone demonstrate a favorable clinical and safety profile to traditional neuroleptics, with particular benefit of olanzapine over risperidone for aspects of quality of life and negative symptoms.

Very few studies have specifically looked at outcome by the age of onset of schizophrenia in late life despite the possibility (as noted above) that the illnesses may be quite different entities. A recent Cochrane Review of the evidence for antipsychotic use in elderly-onset schizophrenia (Arunponpaisal et al, 2004) was unable to find any clinical trials which met their inclusion criteria and was therefore inconclusive. The main reason for exclusion of trials was the inclusion in the study population of both early- and late-onset patients with schizophrenia.

The use of atypical antipsychotics in the elderly (which ideally would be based upon the synthesis of research findings, clinical experience, and evidence from younger populations) has to rely mainly on the latter two influences.

Despite the reality that individual clinical studies in this area have design weaknesses, there is a remarkable consistency of findings between studies (Table 6.2), indicating at least equivalence in terms of efficacy but superiority in terms of EPSE. This alone would certainly argue strongly for the use of atypical antipsychotics as first-line treatment and also serious consideration should be given to switching any elderly patient on a conventional neuroleptic to an atypical drug.

Table 6.2 Summary of evidence to date regarding the use of atypical antipsychotics in elderly patients with schizophrenia

Drug tested	Author(s)	Year	Study design	Sample size	Duration	Key findings
Olanzapine and risperidone	Ritchie*	2004	Open-label, randomized, head-to-head	66	6 months	Olanzapine superior in aspects of QOL and negative symptoms
	Ritchie et al	2003	Open-label, randomized, head-to-head	66	Crossover period (~42 days)	Both improve core symptoms and EPSE. Olanzapine superior in aspects of QOL
	Jeste	2003	Double-blind, randomized, head-to-head	175	8 weeks	, PANSS and EPSE slower to improve with olanzapine. No between-group differences
	Madhusoodanan et al	1999a	Chart review, 37 olanzapine, 114 risperidone	151	N/A	75% olanzapine and 78% risperidone 'responded'. 22% discontinuation risk in both groups and ~16% in each arm developed AE
	Madhusoodanan et al	2000	Prospective cohort	11	Unclear	All showed positive and negative symptom improvement. EPSE in general improved and MMSE and CGI improved in nine of the sample

Drug tested	Author(s)	Year	Study design	Sample size	Duration	Key findings
	Solomons and Geiger	2000	Chart review	58	N/A	60% 'improved' though 38% had an AE noted, which included delirium, EPSE and drowsiness
Olanzapine plus haloperidol	Kennedy et al	2003	Double-blind, randomized	117	6 weeks	Positive symptoms and PANSS total improved with olanzapine more than with haloperidol. Improved akathisia and parkinsonism with olanzapine though no difference in dyskinesia
	Barak et al	2002	Randomized, open-label	20	Unclear	↓PANSS total and negative symptoms subscale better with olanzapine
Risperidone only	Davidson et al	2000	Prospective cohort	180	1 year	54% of sample PANSS by >20% and CGI overall still improving at 1 year. EPSE improved with no spontaneous TD and a decreased use of anticholinergics
	Madhusoodanan et al	1999b	Prospective cohort	103	12 weeks	↓PANSS ↓EPSE
	Kiraly et al	1998	Retrospective elderly vs adult community Rx	112	N/A	Greater efficacy in elderly with lower doses being effective

Drug tested	Author	Year	Study design	Sample size	Duration	Key findings
	Berman et al	1996	Open label dose titration with extension	10	Unclear	↓PANSS total and negative subscale with improved cognitive function noted
Quetiapine only	Tariot	2000	Mixed diagnostic group cohort study	184; 50 with SZ	1 year	13% at baseline had EPSE; parkinsonism but not dyskinesia improved. BPRS and CGI improved with median dose of 137.5 mg
	Madhusoodanan et al	2000	Prospective cohort	7	Unclear	4/7 improved positive symptoms, 3/7 improved negative symptoms and 3/7 had improved EPSE

QOL, quality of life; EPSE, extra-pyramidal side effects; PANSS, positive and negative symptoms score; AE, adverse event; MMSE, Mini-mental State Examination; CGI, clinical global impression; TD, tardive dyskinesia; BPRS, brief psychiatric rating scale; SZ, schizophrenia.

*Unpublished data.

Choosing between atypical neuroleptics

The choice of atypical drug is not clear cut – although most evidence exists for risperidone and olanzapine, which would suggest that one of these two should be the first-line choice.

With regard to safety, the association between both these drugs and stroke in dementia trials (Wooltorton, 2002, 2004) does not seem to apply in elderly patients with schizophrenia, although as the critical evidence in the elderly patient with schizophrenia is scant and of poor quality, it would be wrong to state conclusively that there is no association between these drugs and cerebrovascular compromise.

With regard to movement disorders, it would appear that there is little to choose between any of the atypicals, although as risperidone at higher doses is associated with an increased incidence of EPSE, it may be appropriate to manage patients with existing EPSE or those who are likely to require a higher dose of atypical neuroleptic with olanzapine.

Weight gain is commonly associated with the use of olanzapine in younger populations (Melkersson and Dahl, 2004) – although this side effect is noted to a greater or lesser degree with all neuroleptic drugs. Critical evidence from studies in elderly populations have not noted weight gain to be a major problem, indeed our own study noted that before switching our population had on average quite a low body mass index (BMI) score. We observed a higher average weight gain with olanzapine (although this was not significantly higher than the increase observed with risperidone), which tended to return the average BMI to within the normal range (Ritchie et al, 2003).

Other side effects that have been consistently associated with one or other of the atypical neuroleptics from studies in younger populations include elevation of prolactin (Meaney and O'Keane, 2002) and type 2 diabetes (Wirshing et al, 1998). Although neither of these complications have been conclusively attributed to any one drug it would be wise to monitor blood glucose and prolactin levels in elderly patients on neuroleptics to monitor for the development of type 2 diabetes and the risk of developing osteoporosis.

Conclusions

There is strong evidence which suggests that elderly patients with schizophrenia form a different population to younger people with schizophrenia. Moreover, within this elderly population those individuals with persistent disease from younger adulthood are distinct from those with onset in later life.

Despite this, the evidence base for how to manage these patients from a pharmacological perspective is of very low quality. It is unlikely to improve. Given this, we must base our prescribing on what evidence is available from the elderly and assimilate this with our clinical experience and the high quality evidence from younger populations. This exercise would lead to the conclusion that we should be using atypical antipsychotics in almost all elderly patients with schizophrenia, as the one consistent finding is the reduction of risk for EPSE with this type of drug. Moreover, this side effect is one to which the elderly are particularly susceptible. The choice of which atypical antipsychotic to use is less clear.

It is unlikely that expensive, high quality, large clinical trials will be conducted to help answer which atypical drug is better in particular circumstances – although on the basis of the evidence to date, any particular advantage of one drug over the other is likely to be small.

References

Arunponpaisal S, Ahmed I, Aqueel N et al, Antipsychotic drug treatment for elderly people with late-onset schizophrenia (Cochrane Dementia and Cognitive Improvement Group). In: *The Cochrane Library* (John Wiley & Sons: Chichester, UK, 2004).

Barak Y, Shamir E, Zemishlani H et al, Olanzapine vs. haloperidol in the treatment of elderly chronic schizophrenia patients, *Prog Neuropsychopharmacol Biol Psychiatry* (2002) **26**:1199–202.

Berman I, Merson A, Rachov-Pavlov J et al, Risperidone in elderly schizophrenic patients, *Am J Geriatric Psychiatry* (1996) **4**:173–8.

Brown S, Excess mortality of schizophrenia, *Br J Psychiatry* (1997) **171**:502–8.

Bullmore ET, Frangou S, Murray RM, The dysplastic net hypothesis: an integration of developmental and dysconnectivity theories of schizophrenia, *Schizophr Res* (1997) **28**:143–56.

Burns A, Förstl H, Neuropathological and neuroradiological correlates of paranoid symptoms in organic mental disorders, *Eur Arch Psychiatr Clin Neurosci* (1997) **247**:190–4.

Davidson M, Harvey PD, Vervacke J et al, A long-term, multicentre, open-label study of risperidone in elderly patients with psychosis, *Int J Geriatr Psychiatry* (2000) **15**:506–14.

Geddes J, Freemantle N, Harrison P, Bebbington P, Atypical antipsychotics in the treatment of schizophrenia: systematic overview and meta-regression, *BMJ* (2000) **321**:1371–6.

Jeste DV, Barak Y, Madhusoodanan S et al, International multisite double-blind trial of the atypical antipsychotics risperidone and olanzapine in 175 elderly patients with chronic schizophrenia, *Am J Geriatr Psychiatry* (2003) **11**:638–47.

Jeste DV, Caligiuri MP, Paulsen JS et al, Risk of tardive dyskinesia in older patients: a prospective longitudinal study of 266 patients, *Arch Gen Psychiatry* (1995) **52**:756–65.

Jeste DV, Rockwell E, Harris MJ et al, Conventional versus newer antipsychotics in elderly, *Am J Geriatric Psychiatry* (1999) **7**:70–6.

Joshi PM, Joshi U, Risperidone in treatment-resistant geriatric patients with chronic psychosis and concurrent medical illnesses. In: Abstracts of the *149th Annual Meeting of the American Psychiatric Association*, New York, USA, May 4–9 (1996) Abstract NR337.

Kennedy JS, Jeste D, Kaiser CJ et al, Olanzapine vs haloperidol in geriatric schizophrenia: analysis of data from a double-blind controlled trial, *Int J Geriatr Psychiatry* (2003) **18**:1013–20.

Kiraly SJ, Gibson RE, Ancill RJ, Holliday SG, Risperidone: treatment response in adult and geriatric patients, *Int J Psychiatry Med* (1998) **28**:255–63.

Madhusoodanan S, Brenner R, Kascow JW et al, Risperidone in elderly patients with psychotic disorders. In: New Research Program and Abstracts of the *150th Annual Meeting of the American Psychiatric Association*, San Diego, USA, May 18, 1997 (1999b) Abstract NR601:230.

Madhusoodanan S, Brenner R, Suresh P et al, Efficacy and tolerability of olanzapine in elderly patients with psychotic disorders: a prospective study, *Ann Clin Psychiatry* (2000) **12**:11–18.

Madhusoodanan S, Brenner R, Araujo L, Abaza A, Efficacy of risperidone treatment for psychoses associated with schizophrenia, schizoaffective disorder, bipolar disorder, or senile dementia in 11 geriatric patients: a case series, *J Clin Psychiatry* (1995) **56**:514–18.

Madhusoodanan S, Suresh P, Brenner R, Pillai R, Experience with the atypical antipsychotics risperidone and olanzapine in the elderly, *Ann Clin Psychiatry* (1999a) **11**:113–18.

Meaney AM, O'Keane V, Prolactin and schizophrenia: clinical consequences of hyperprolactinaemia, *Life Sci* (2002) **71**:979–92.

Melkersson K, Dahl ML, Adverse metabolic effects associated with atypical antipsychotics: literature review and clinical implications, *Drugs* (2004) **64**:701–23.

Miller BL, Lesser IM, Boone KB et al, Brain lesions and cognitive function in late life psychosis, *Br J Psychiatry* (1991) **158**:76–82.

Ritchie CW, Chiu E, Harrigan S et al, The impact upon extra-pyramidal side effects, clinical symptoms and quality of life of a switch from conventional to atypical antipsychotics (risperidone or olanzapine) in elderly patients with schizophrenia, *Int J Geriatr Psychiatry* (2003) **18**:432–40.

Roth M, Kay DWK, Late paraphrenia: a variant of schizophrenia manifest in late life or an organic clinical syndrome? A review of recent evidence, *Int J Geriatr Psychiatry* (1998) **13**:1013–20.

Solomons K, Geiger O, Olanzapine use in the elderly: a retrospective analysis, *Can J Psychiatry* (2000) **45**:151–5.

Sweet RA, Pollock BG, Neuroleptics in the elderly: guidelines for monitoring, *Harvard Rev Psychiatry* (1995) 2:327–35.

Tariot PN, Salzman C, Yeung PP et al, Long-term use of quetiapine in elderly patients with psychotic disorders, *Clin Ther* (2000) **22**:1068–84.

Weinberger DR, Implications of normal brain development for the pathogenesis of schizophrenia, *Arch Gen Psychiatry* (1987) **44**:660–9.

Wirshing DA, Spellberg BJ, Lanzio M et al, Novel antipsychotics and new onset diabetes, *Biol Psychiatry* (1998) **44**:778–83.

Wooltorton E, Risperidone (Risperdal): increase rate of cerebrovascular events in dementia trials, *Can Med Assoc J* (2002) **167**:1269–70.

Wooltorton E, Olanzapine (Zyprexa): increase rate of cerebrovascular events in dementia trials, *Can Med Assoc J* (2004) **170**:1395.

chapter 7

Psychosocial rehabilitation of the elderly with early- or late-onset schizophrenia: general principles

Vincent Camus and Carlos Augusto de Mendonça-Lima

Introduction

Schizophrenia is one of the mental disorders that has the most severe consequences in terms of psychosocial functioning. Pharmacological treatments
have been shown to have a more significant impact on positive symptoms of
the disease, while negative symptoms, functional and social disability, as well
as everyday functioning in the community, have been defined as the main
targets of psychosocial rehabilitation programs. On the other hand, aging by
itself may constitute a risk of functional decline, particularly in the last two
years of life (Covinsky et al, 2003), or in the case of very advanced age (Hebert
et al, 1997), or severe medical co-morbidity such as hypertension, cerebrovascular disease, arthritis (McCurry et al, 2002) or cognitive decline
(Nyenhuis et al, 2002). Preservation of strong social relations has also been
reported to have a significant protective impact against disability in aging
(Avlund et al, 2004). Elderly people suffering from schizophrenia are both
aged patients with a lifelong evolution of early-onset schizophrenia, and
patients suffering from what has been recently termed as 'late-onset schizophrenia' (a psychotic disorder occurring between the ages of 40 and 60) and
'very-late-onset schizophrenia-like psychosis' (a psychotic disorder occurring

after the age of 60) (Howard et al, 2000). Because of their advanced age, their potential somatic co-morbidity, and some specific clinical and social aspects of schizophrenia, like delusions, misinterpretations, cognitive dysfunction, and social isolation (Hassett, 1999), they are also particularly exposed to functional and social disability. Psychosocial rehabilitation has been developed during the past decades in parallel with pharmacological treatments, so as to offer a more comprehensive approach of psychiatric care in a range of psychiatric disorders, including schizophrenia. Their use in aged schizophrenic patients needs to take into account some specificities of both clinical and social aspects of schizophrenia in advanced age, and of organization of care for elderly people suffering from mental disorders.

Psychosocial rehabilitation: general principles

Historical perspective

The concept of rehabilitation progressively emerged in the late 1940s and early 1950s, when European and American societies had to deal with a large number of physically disabled veterans because of war injuries. At the same time, the de-institutionalization movement pressed mental health professionals to experiment with new techniques for improving community-based continued care and social integration of chronic psychiatric patients. Considering that the goals of psychiatric care are not limited to achieving an attenuation of the symptoms of the disorder, efforts have been directed to improving the social adaptation of patients. Beyond these objectives, ultimate goals of the care process are also to try to improve quality of life, to enhance patient satisfaction, to alleviate the family burden, and finally to improve caregiver satisfaction (Bertolote, 1993). In a such perspective, psychiatric rehabilitation has progressively become a complementary approach to pharmacological management and psychotherapy in the long-term care of patients suffering from chronic mental disorders.

Current definitions

Disability and handicap

As it has been shown that diagnosis alone does not confidently predict service needs, length of hospitalization, level of care or functional outcomes, the current classification system that has been elaborated by the World Health Organization (WHO) proposes to distinguish symptoms and etiologies of the psychiatric disorders (International Classification of Diseases, 10th revision,

ICD-10) (WHO, 1992) from the description of level of individual functioning (International Classification of Functioning, Disability and Health, ICF) (WHO, 2001). The previous version of the WHO International Classification of Impairments, Disabilities, and Handicaps (ICIDH) (WHO, 1980) was mostly a 'consequence of diseases' classification, focusing on the impact of the disease on the body or physiologic function, on personal limitations, and on their social consequences. In that perspective, *impairment* was defined as any loss or abnormality of psychological, physiological or anatomical structure or function; a *disability* as any restriction or lack (resulting from an impairment) of ability to perform an activity in the manner or within the range considered normal for a human being; a *handicap* as a disadvantage for a given individual, resulting from an impairment or a disability, and that prevents the fulfillment of a role that is considered normal (depending on age, sex and social and cultural factors) for that individual. The current ICF has moved toward a 'components of health' classification. It refers to two main categories of descriptors: functioning and disability, and contextual factors. Functioning and disabilities have two components: body structures and functions, and activities and participation. Both can be expressed in positive or negative terms (functional and structural impairments or integrity, activity limitations or participation). Contextual factors describe the complete personal environmental and social context. This shift from a reference to impairments, disabilities, and handicaps towards the concepts of functioning, disability, and health has probably facilitated the evolution of concepts of psychiatric rehabilitation (WHO, 1995).

Rehabilitation

To 'rehabilitate' has several meanings: (1) to restore a former rank, right, privilege, that has been lost; (2) to restore to a previous health condition; (3) to restore to a useful and constructive place in society. According to this definition – and in reference to the previous WHO approach of impairments, disabilities, and handicaps – rehabilitation has been initially defined as the process that limits disabilities through skills development, compensates disabilities by providing a supportive environment, and fights stigma and discrimination that increase the social handicap of a mentally ill individual. Rather than focusing on deficits, the rehabilitation process takes advantage of residual functional and social capabilities that were spared by the illness. Therefore, it contributes to maintaining and preventing secondary disability, to recovery in terms of symptomatology, resettlement in job activity and to improving social integration (Burti and Yastrebov, 1993).

The recent evolution of the International Classification of Impairments, Disabilities and Handicaps (ICIDH) towards the International Classification of Functioning, Disability and Health (ICF) has given a new framework for understanding disability and functioning. These have been proposed to be expressed in a dialectic of 'medical model' versus 'social model'. The medical model views disability as a feature of the person, directly caused by disease, trauma or other health condition, which requires medical care provided in the form of individual treatment by professionals. Disability, on this model, calls for medical or other treatment or intervention, to 'correct' the problem with the individual. On the other hand, the social model considers disability as a socially created problem and not at all an attribute of an individual. On the social model, disability demands a political response, since the problem is created by an unaccommodating physical environment brought about by attitudes and other features of the social environment. In this perspective, the management of the problem requires social action and political determination by planning the environmental adjustments that are needed for a full integration of people with disabilities. On their own, neither model is adequate, although both are partially valid. The current concept of psychosocial rehabilitation is deeply rooted in this comprehensive view and construct of health through a biological, individual, and social perspective.

The current concept of psychosocial rehabilitation

A consensus statement recently proposed by a joint initiative of the WHO and the World Association for Psychosocial Rehabilitation (WAPR), has defined psychosocial rehabilitation as 'a process that facilitates the opportunity for individuals – who are impaired, disabled or handicapped by a mental disorder – to reach their optimal level of independent functioning in the community. It implies both improving individuals' competencies and introducing environmental changes in order to create a life of the best quality possible for people who have experienced a mental disorder, or who have an impairment of their mental capacity which produces a certain level of disability' (WHO, 1995). In this perspective, psychosocial rehabilitation tends to achieve several complementary objectives: (1) reducing symptomatology through appropriate pharmacological or psychotherapeutic treatments; (2) reducing iatrogenesis by limiting medical and social adverse effects of therapeutic interventions; (3) improving social competence by enhancing social skills, psychological coping, and occupational functioning; (4) reducing discrimination and stigma; (5) providing support to those families with a member with a mental disorder; (6) providing social support by creating and maintaining a long-term system of social support covering basic needs related to housing, employment, leisure; (7) enhancing consumer's and carer's autonomy, self-sufficiency, and self-advocacy. Consequently, psychosocial rehabilitation hinges on three different levels of operation: the individual level, the mental health services' level, and the societal level. The main components of intervention are as follows. (1) At the individual level: pharmacological treatment, independent living and social skills training, psychological support and treatment to patients and their families, housing, vocational rehabilitation and employment, social support networking, leisure. (2) At the mental health services' level: mental health service policy and fund allocation, improvement of institutional and residential settings, training for staff, quality assurance. (3) At the societal level: improvement of pertinent legislation, consumer empowerment, improvement of public opinion and attitudes related to mental disorders, fighting stigma and discrimination (WHO, 1995). In such a perspective, psychiatric rehabilitation is not solely targeted to tertiary prevention by limiting the consequences of the chronic mental disease, but in an additional major effort to improve the patient's quality of life from the earliest manifestations of the disease (Cancro, 2002).

Psychosocial rehabilitation in various psychiatric conditions

Psychosocial rehabilitation has been experienced in several types of mental disorders, but its main scope has been mostly limited to severe mental illnesses, such as schizophrenia (Fenton and Schooler, 2000) or substance abuse disorders with or without co-morbid psychiatric states (Drake and Mueser, 2000). In schizophrenia, psychosocial rehabilitation has been experienced through several types of specific interventions such as family psychoeducation programs (Dixon et al, 2000), family therapy (Langsley et al, 1993), practical and emotional support to patients and their caregivers (Fenton, 2000), and social skills training (Liberman, 1988). Nevertheless the level of implementation of these techniques seems to be strongly dependent on the ability of the local care system to integrate them into basic community-based care (Lehman, 2000).

Psychosocial rehabilitation in old age psychiatry

One of the recent textbooks in old age psychiatry defines the main goals of rehabilitation for older people suffering from mental disorders as: (1)

restoring and maintaining the highest possible level of psychological, physical, and social function despite the disabling effects of illness; (2) preventing unnecessary handicap associated with illness or secondary to maladaptive responses to illness; (3) combating the deadening effects of low expectations of older people among patients, families, and society in general (Jones, 2002). Considering the contribution of the recent ICF, it could be added that psychosocial rehabilitation in old age can be considered as the set of direct or indirect processes by which an aged individual with impairment or disability from a mental disorder can recover an optimal level of activities and participation (de Mendonça-Lima et al, 2003). In their initial consensus statement on the definition of old age psychiatry, the WHO and the World Psychiatric Association (WPA) stated that objectives of treatment in old age psychiatry may include restoration of health, but also improvement of quality of life, minimization of disability, preservation of autonomy, and attention to supporters' needs. They emphasized the necessity to deliver care in a multidisciplinary way, involving the widest range of professionals and nonprofessionals, to provide therapeutic interventions that should encourage autonomy by including retraining in daily living skills, improving safety at home, providing practical support including social and legal rights' advice (WPA/WHO, 1996). In their second consensus statement on organization of care in old age psychiatry, they added that a coherent and a comprehensive care plan should address both the individual's physical, psychological, social, spiritual, and material needs, as well as the needs of the carer network (WPA/WHO, 1997). These general principles of care in old age psychiatry are congruent with those of psychiatric rehabilitation, as mentioned above, and show how old age psychiatry integrates the holistic approach that characterizes psychosocial rehabilitation.

Main strategies in psychosocial rehabilitation for elderly patients suffering from schizophrenia

Although psychosis in the elderly has received less attention than other diseases in terms of clinical research in old age psychiatry, there are now some specific data on its clinical characterization, outcome, and treatment. Some of these data account for emerging evidence on how to develop psychosocial rehabilitation for elderly patients suffering from schizophrenia at the individual level, mental health resources level, and societal level.

The individual level

The first type of intervention at the individual level is pharmacological treatment see Chapter 6). Atypical antipsychotics have been demonstrated to be at least as efficacious as conventional antipsychotics, with a better safety and tolerability profile (Sable and Jeste, 2003), particularly in terms of extrapyramidal symptoms and of risk of incidence of tardive dyskinesia (Woerner et al, 1998; Jeste et al, 1999). That could explain why their use seems to be associated with a better adherence; even so the overall compliance rate is rather low (about 55% at 12 months) (Dolder et al, 2002). Interestingly, adherence to medication has been shown to be correlated with cognitive disturbances in older outpatients with schizophrenia (Jeste et al, 2003). Various types of cognitive and neuropsychological deficits including executive functions, short-term, working or declarative memory, and motor ability have been described as clinical features of both acute phase (Sullivan et al, 1994) and remission phase (Nuechterlein and Dawson, 1984) of schizophrenia in young adults, and seem to be preferentially associated with negative symptoms (Nieuwenstein et al, 2001). Neurocognitive dysfunctions have been described in elderly schizophrenic patients as well (Harvey et al, 1995). These deficits are strongly correlated with negative symptomatology, overall functional status and specific adaptive deficits (Harvey et al, 1998; Patterson et al, 1998; Twamley et al, 2002). Psychological management of the elderly patient with psychosis is another major component of the intervention at the individual level, ranging from a standard home or outpatient clinic visit to formal psychotherapy (Aguera Ortiz and Reneses Prieto, 2003). As now well established in young adults, the effectiveness of social skills training programs for elderly patients suffering from schizophrenia is beginning to be tested. Preliminary results state that such an approach has good feasibility and arouses good adherence (McQuaid et al, 2000), with encouraging results.

The mental health resources level

As mentioned in the WHO/WAPR consensus statement (WHO, 1995), psychosocial rehabilitation should be considered as an essential component in every mental health service policy. Particularly, in such a perspective, community-based mental health services should be 'case manager centers' able not only to provide treatment but also to facilitate access to community resources for patients and their relatives. A high level of use of community support services has been reported by elderly patients with psychotic disorders living in an urban area of the United States (California). But the frequency of contact with community care facilities was related to some clinical characteristics of the patients. In particular, the presence of more severe and negative symptoms was associated with a lower rate of referral (Shaw et al, 2000). And apart from clinical characteristics, the local level of development of the community care system probably has a major impact on access to care. Even in the UK where the mental health care system is strongly community-based oriented with a supposed facilitated accessibility, it seems that many care needs of elderly schizophrenic patients are not covered or are only partially covered (McNulty et al, 2003). Keeping in mind that the level of development of specific services in old age psychiatry is very limited in most countries (Reifler and Cohen, 1998), we can assume that results from the UK are more the rule rather than an exception throughout the world (see Chapter 8). This underlies how the specific needs of elderly patients must be taken into account in the development of mental health policies and services (WPA/WHO, 1997), and how both types of mental disorders including schizophrenia have to be addressed in specific training programs aimed at the full range of professionals (Camus et al, 2003). Finally, setting up living alternatives to the mental hospital has been defined as a major component of psychosocial rehabilitation. In fact, as a consequence of the de-institutionalization movement, many middle-aged and aged schizophrenic patients have been admitted into nursing homes (Harvey et al, 1998). But patients in residential settings are the most severely impaired in terms of cognitive function and severity of symptomatology (Gupta et al, 2003). As a consequence of that, specialized care has to be given in residential settings, whose professional carers should be trained and supported by old age psychiatry or mental health care teams (see Chapter 9).

The societal level

The stigma attached to mental disorders affects not only patients suffering from these disorders, but also carers – both family members and health workers. Negative opinions of the general population concerning severe mental illness contribute to the social isolation and distress of patients (Crisp et al, 2000). This stigmatization, by its harmful effect on patients' self-esteem, increases their social withdrawal and handicap (Link et al, 2001). Destigmatization of people with mental disorders has become a major concern of WHO and WPA, but most action has been focused on young adults, particularly those suffering from schizophrenia (Sartorius, 1997; Gaebel and

Baumann, 2003). More recently, the urgent need for specific actions for fighting stigma and preventing discrimination among elderly people suffering from mental disorders has been pointed out, since stigma against old age adds to that against mental disorder, constituting a 'double jeopardy' for older people with mental disorders (Graham et al, 2003). As schizophrenia is one of the most stigmatizing diseases, schizophrenia in old age needs some specific and targeted actions to reduce its stigmatizing effect (see Chapter 10).

Concluding remarks

Because psychiatry of the elderly has emerged more recently in the field of mental health care, many specific actions and care processes initially developed in adult psychiatry have been experienced and implemented later in the field of old age psychiatry. In this perspective, we have to particularly review any efforts suggesting that aged schizophrenic patients could benefit from psychosocial rehabilitation techniques that have been demonstrated to be effective in adulthood (i.e. social skills training programs). Nevertheless, the journey from clinical experimentation by very specialized and research teams to actual clinical practice by first-line professionals in the real world would require considerable committed efforts (Lehman, 2000). Indeed specific research on how to improve care processes in psychosocial rehabilitation for aged schizophrenic patients must be encouraged. In parallel, efforts have to be maintained to promote the development and implementation of policies, programs, and services in old age psychiatry. As services in old age psychiatry have been recommended to be strongly community-based and multidisciplinary, a psychosocial rehabilitation approach should be embedded into its development and practice.

References

Aguera Ortiz L, Reneses Prieto B, Practical psychological management of old age psychosis, *J Nutr Health Aging* (2003) 7:412–20.

Avlund K, Lund R, Holstein BE, Due P, Social relations as determinant of onset of disability in aging, *Arch Gerontol Geriatr* (2004) **38**:85–99.

Bertolote JM, Quality assurance in mental health. In: Sartorius N, De Girolamo G, Andrews GA et al, eds, *Treatment of Mental Disorders. A Review of Effectiveness* (American Psychiatric Association: Washington DC, 1993) 443–61.

Burti L, Yastrebov VS, Procedures used in rehabilitation. In: Sartorius N, De Girolamo G, Andrews GA et al, eds, *Treatment of Mental Disorders. A Review of Effectiveness* (American Psychiatric Association: Washington DC, 1993) 289–336.

Camus V, Katona C, Mendonca Lima CA et al, Teaching and training in old age psychiatry: a general survey of the World Psychiatric Association member societies, *Int J Geriat Psychiatry* (2003) **18**:694–9.

Cancro R, Psychiatric rehabilitation. In: Christodoulou GN, ed, *Recent Advances in Psychiatry* (Betha Medical Publishers: Athens, 2002) 1141–5.

Covinsky KE, Eng C, Lui LY et al, The last 2 years of life: functional trajectories of frail older people, *J Am Geriatr Soc* (2003) **51**:492–8.

Crisp AH, Gelder MG, Rix S et al, Stigmatisation of people with mental illnesses, *Br J Psychiatry* (2000) **177**:4–7.

de Mendonça-Lima CA, Kühne N, Bertolote JM, Camus V, Psychose, réadaptation psychosociale, psychiatrie de la personne âgée: concepts et principes généraux, *L'Année Gérontologique* (2003) **17**:347–68.

Dixon L, Adams C, Lucksted A, Update on family psychoeducation for schizophrenia, *Schizophr Bull* (2000) **26**:5–20.

Dolder CR, Lacro JP, Dunn LB, Jeste DV, Antipsychotic medication adherence: is there a difference between typical and atypical agents?, *Am J Psychiatry* (2002) **159**:103–8.

Drake RE, Mueser KT, Psychosocial approaches to dual diagnosis, *Schizophr Bull* (2000) **26**:105–18.

Fenton WS, Evolving perspectives on individual psychotherapy for schizophrenia, *Schizophr Bull* (2000) **26**:47–72.

Fenton WS, Schooler NR, Evidence-based psychosocial treatment for schizophrenia, *Schizophr Bull* (2000) **26**:1–3.

Gaebel W, Baumann AE, Interventions to reduce the stigma associated with severe mental illness: experiences from the open the doors program in Germany, *Can J Psychiatry* (2003) **48**:657–62.

Graham N, Katona CLE, Lindesay J et al, Reducing stigma and discrimination against older people with mental disorders: a technical consensus statement, *Int J Geriatr Psychiatry* (2003) **18**:678.

Gupta S, Steinmeyer C, Frank B et al, Older patients with schizophrenia: nature of dwelling status and symptom severity, *Am J Psychiatry* (2003) **160**:383–4.

Harvey PD, Howanitz E, Parrella M et al, Symptoms, cognitive functioning, and adaptive skills in geriatric patients with lifelong schizophrenia: a comparison across treatment sites, *Am J Psychiatry* (1998) **155**:1080–6.

Harvey PD, Powchik P, Mohs RC, Davidson M, Memory functions in geriatric chronic schizophrenic patients: a neuropsychological study, *J Neuropsychiatry Clin Neurosci* (1995) **7**:207–12.

Hassett A, A descriptive study of first presentation of psychosis in old age, *Aust N Z J Psychiatry* (1999) **33**:814–24.

Hebert R, Brayne C, Spiegelhalter D, Incidence of functional decline and improvement in a community-dwelling, very elderly population, *Am J Epidemiol* (1997) **145**:935–44.

Howard R, Rabins PV, Seeman MV, Jeste DV, Late-onset schizophrenia and very-late-onset schizophrenia-like psychosis: an international consensus. The International Late-Onset Schizophrenia Group, *Am J Psychiatry* (2000) **157**:172–8.

Jeste DV, Lacro JP, Palmer B et al, Incidence of tardive dyskinesia in early stages of low-dose treatment with typical neuroleptics in older patients, *Am J Psychiatry* (1999) **156**:309–11.

Jeste SD, Patterson TL, Palmer BW et al, Cognitive predictors of medication adherence among middle-aged and older outpatients with schizophrenia, *Schizophr Res* (2003) **63**:49–58.

Jones R, Rehabilitation. In: Copeland JRM, Abou-Saleh MT, Blazer DG, eds, *Principles and Practices of Geriatric Psychiatry*, 2nd edn (John Wiley & Sons: Chichester 2002) 739–42.

Langsley DG, Hodes M, Grimson WR, Psychosocial interventions. In: Sartorius N, De Girolamo G, Andrews GA et al, eds, *Treatment of Mental Disorders. A Review of Effectiveness* (American Psychiatric Association: Washington DC, 1993) 253–88.

Lehman AF, Commentary: what happens to psychosocial treatments on the way to the clinic?, *Schizophr Bull* (2000) 26:137–9.

Liberman RP, *Psychiatric Rehabilitation of Chronic Mental Patients* (American Psychiatric Association: Washington, DC, 1988).

Link BG, Struening EL, Neese-Todd S et al, Stigma as a barrier to recovery: the consequences of stigma for the self-esteem of people with mental illnesses, *Psychiatr Serv* (2001) 52:1621–6.

McCurry SM, Gibbons LE, Bond GE et al, Older adults and functional decline: a cross-cultural comparison, *Int Psychogeriatr* (2002) 14:161–79.

McNulty SV, Duncan L, Semple M et al, Care needs of elderly people with schizophrenia: assessment of an epidemiologically defined cohort in Scotland, *Br J Psychiatry* (2003) 182:241–7.

McQuaid JR, Granholm E, McClure FS et al, Development of an integrated cognitive-behavioral and social skills training intervention for older patients with schizophrenia, *J Psychother Pract Res* (2000) 9:149–56.

Nieuwenstein MR, Aleman A, de Haan EH, Relationship between symptom dimensions and neurocognitive functioning in schizophrenia: a meta-analysis of WCST and CPT studies. Wisconsin Card Sorting Test. Continuous Performance Test, *J Psychiatr Res* (2001) 35:119–25.

Nuechterlein KH, Dawson ME, Information processing and attentional functioning in the developmental course of schizophrenic disorders, *Schizophr. Bull* (1984) 10:160–203.

Nyenhuis DL, Gorelick PB, Freels S, Garron DC, Cognitive and functional decline in African Americans with VaD, AD, and stroke without dementia, *Neurology* (2002) 58:56–61.

Patterson TL, Klapow JC, Eastham JH et al, Correlates of functional status in older patients with schizophrenia, *Psychiatry Res* (1998) 80:41–52.

Reifler BV, Cohen W, Practice of geriatric psychiatry and mental health services for the elderly: results of an international survey, *Int Psychogeriatr* (1998) 10:351–7.

Sable JA, Jeste DV, Pharmacologic management of psychosis in the elderly, *J Nutr Health Aging* (2003) 7:421–7.

Sartorius N, Fighting schizophrenia and its stigma. A new World Psychiatric Association educational programme, *Br J Psychiatry* (1997) 170:297.

Shaw WS, Patterson TL, Semple SJ et al, Use of community support services by middle-aged and older patients with psychotic disorders, *Psychiatr Serv* (2000) 51:506–12.

Sullivan EV, Shear PK, Zipursky RB et al, A deficit profile of executive, memory, and motor functions in schizophrenia, *Biol Psychiatry* (1994) 36:641–53.

Twamley EW, Doshi RR, Nayak GV et al, Generalized cognitive impairments, ability to perform everyday tasks, and level of independence in community living situations of older patients with psychosis, *Am J Psychiatry* (2002) 159:2013–20.

World Health Organization *WHO International Classification of Impairments, Disabilities, and Handicaps: A Manual of Classification Relating to the Consequences of Disease* (*WHO*: Geneva, 1980).

World Health Organization *WHO International Classification of Diseases and Related Health Problems*, 10th revision (*WHO*: Geneva, 1992).

World Health Organization *WHO Psychosocial Rehabilitation: A Consensus Statement (DOC: WHO/MNH/MND/96.2)* (*WHO*: Geneva, 1995).

World Health Organization *WHO International Classification of Functioning, Disability, and Health* (*WHO*: Geneva, 2001).

Woerner MG, Alvir JM, Saltz BL et al, Prospective study of tardive dyskinesia in the elderly: rates and risk factors, *Am J Psychiatry* (1998) **155**:1521–8.

World Psychiatric Association/World Health Organization *WPA/WHO Psychiatry of the Elderly: A Consensus Statement (DOC: WHO/MNH/MND/96.7) (World Health Organization*: Geneva, 1996).

World Psychiatric Association/World Health Organization *WPA/WHO Organisation of Care in Psychiatry of the Elderly: a Technical Consensus Statement (DOC: WHO/MSA/MNH/MND/97.3) (World Health Organization*: Geneva, 1997).

chapter 8

A multidisciplinary approach to community-based long-term care for older people with early- or late-onset schizophrenia

Rosemary Kelleher, Lina Gibson, Amanda Carter and Catherine Waterhouse

What is multidisciplinary community-based long-term care?

Multidisciplinary community-based long-term care consists of a range of specialized services – usually delivered by a publicly funded mental health service – which are free of charge to patients with serious and continuing mental health problems. A clinical member of staff, known as a case manager, is given responsibility for looking after the treatment and support needs of a limited number of patients. The case manager has a professional training in the delivery of community mental health services, and may be a social worker, psychiatric nurse, occupational therapist, psychologist, neuropsychologist or psychiatrist (Metropolitan Health and Aged Care Services Division, 2002a). A team of case managers functions under the supervision of a consultant psychiatrist.

The goal of multidisciplinary community-based long-term care is to maximize the patient's ability to live independently in the community with the best possible quality of life. An individual service plan is developed and documented by the case manager and the client together. This written summary of treatment goals and the strategies by which they will be achieved covers many aspects of the patient's health, social support and spiritual needs. The plan is written in a way that can easily be understood by the patient, family members, and carers.

Community-based long-term care may be delivered over an extended period beyond the acute episode that may have precipitated the referral. Subsequent acute episodes may be managed proactively, often either avoiding acute admissions or reducing the length of admission and the attendant social disruption to client and family that may otherwise occur. National Standards are established for such services in Australia (Commonwealth of Australia, 1996).

Current thinking about community-based services for older people with schizophrenia

Current thinking supports a multifaceted approach to planning and delivering care for people with schizophrenia, and calls for more age-specific research into the effectiveness of various treatment modalities.

A review of current studies of community-based treatment for people with severe psychiatric disorders provides some pointers for program development for people over 65 years of age with a diagnosis of schizophrenia (Mohamed et al, 2003). Program models reviewed included assertive community treatment, case management, vocational rehabilitation, supported housing, day treatment, and client clubhouses. Deficient sampling of older people, however, limited the potential to analyse day and clubhouse programs' potential to meet the needs of older people with schizophrenia. Similarly, only provisional assessment of the likely benefits of assertive community treatment for this population could be undertaken.

The researchers reviewed 20 studies of a range of case management models. Case management was broadly defined as support provided for patients as they negotiate for the different services they desire (Mohamed et al, 2003, p.207). Of the 20 programs reviewed, eight included persons aged 50 and over. Positive or mixed outcomes were reported in six of these eight programs. Case management appears to be most beneficial for older persons who lack involved caregivers and are living alone in the community (Mohamed et al, 2003, p.210). Kilian et al developed an interesting framework for examining how urban-dwelling people aged 18 to 65 with severe and persistent schizophrenia perceive their level of social integration, and

how particular types of social integration are related to the use of day centers and patient clubs in Leipzig, Germany (Kilian et al, 2001). This framework would also merit application for patients over 65 years of age with a
corresponding diagnosis.

Few if any advantages of vocational rehabilitation have been found among
an older population (see Mohamed et al, 2003, pp.211–12). Several studies,
however, show that volunteerism among older people in the general population has potential benefits of improved life satisfaction, self-esteem and
mood. Mohamed et al suggest, in the absence of any known research, that
volunteerism may be an under-used option for people with schizophrenia
(Mohammed et al, 2003, p.213). Research by Spaid (1998, pp.24–30) supports
this view, finding that there were no differences in giving or receiving instrumental or expressive social supports regardless of whether the respondents
were diagnosed with a chronic mental illness. Our work with the cohort
described below also supports the notion that people with chronic mental illness have – or can be assisted to nurture – social connections. The potential
benefits of social support groups for older people with schizophrenia merit
further exploration and documentation.

Older people with schizophrenia use about the same level of social services
and daily living services as people with Alzheimer's disease. This may suggest
that there are benefits in changing from treating symptoms to increasing
social well-being in older people with schizophrenia (Shaw et al, 2000).
Mohamed et al strongly advocate more research into this population, especially to establish whether existing programs can be adapted to meet their
needs, or whether alternative programs would better serve the specific health,
cognitive and functional adaptive abilities of older people with schizophrenia
(Mohammed et al, 2003, p.219).

An innovative service response to high-risk older people with schizophrenia, dementia, and depression who are considered unlikely to self-refer for
mental health services is documented by Raschko (1998). In this outreach
program a wide range of people, from gas meter readers to public transport
system drivers, are trained to identify older people in the community at risk
of mental health problems. The program then provides interdisciplinary evaluation, planning, support, co-ordination, and advocacy services, including a
24–hour crisis intervention service. This is one of very few studies specifically
considering the service access needs of older people with recent onset of late
paraphrenia. The capacity for relationship building is considered an essential

skill for workers on this program. It is also a significant requirement for workers in community-based long-term care for older people with schizophrenia.

The application of the multidisciplinary approach in the community

A multidisciplinary approach to long-term community-based care carries with it complex choices for patients and for workers. There are dilemmas in relation to therapeutic engagement, modes of service delivery, and the timing of the application of statutory responsibilities. There is a delicate course to chart between individual liberty on the one hand and, on the other, the safety and well-being of the patient and those around them. Any application of statutory interventions should be the least restrictive alternative. Secure leadership and personal and professional trust within the multidisciplinary team can help workers from all disciplines contribute to the best service for the more vulnerable statutory patients and their carers.

In this chapter, we draw on our experience as members of a multidisciplinary team of an Aged Persons Mental Health Service (APMHS) providing community-based long-term care in inner suburban Melbourne, Australia. We present some data on 22 patients who have used our service, and discuss in detail one man with late-onset schizophrenia and one woman patient with early-onset schizophrenia. These case examples demonstrate the complexity of the work and the benefits of long-term multidisciplinary community-based work with older clients.

Bearing in mind the principle of the 'least restrictive alternative', many services do not incorporate continuing care into their model of service delivery. Without a continuing care component for some patients, however, the service model is based on crisis intervention and minimum service. Long-term mental illness reaching into old age impacts on multiple aspects of the person's emotional, clinical, social, and economic well-being. Continuing care – where possible establishing strong links with mainstream community agencies – monitors the patient through the course of the illness, from the acute to the more stable phase, reducing the risk of relapse. Whilst this may constitute a longer period of engagement with the client, we observe anecdotally that there is a significant reduction of relapse once they have been discharged from the service.

We have reviewed a selected sample of 22 people aged between 65 and 87 (10 male, 12 female; mean age at time of referral to APMHS = 70.2, median age = 70) with early- or late-onset schizophrenia who have received community-based long-term care from our service. All these people received case management and had complex care needs. Three men and three women in the cohort were also involved in rehabilitation group programs. Statutory patients are a particularly vulnerable group – although most, through long-term case management, have come to accept the caseworkers in their lives so no longer require a Community Treatment Order (CTO).[1] Of the cohort, six were placed on CTOs at the time of discharge from the inpatient unit; four of these people have since been discharged from their involuntary status as a result of long-term case management. More generally, of the 22 long-term patients in the cohort, 12 (54.5%, five men, seven women) were successfully discharged from the service altogether after a period of case management by our service.

Many patients were living independently in the community at the time of referral to our service. Four males and six females were independent in self-care, of whom one male and two females living independently in the community received home care services from the local municipal council at the time of referral to the APMHS. One male and one female accepted referrals to home care and/or personal care services. Six men and four women living independently refused home care and/or personal care services which case managers would have considered to be appropriate supports. Of these, two men and three women were living in domestic squalor at the time of referral.

Patients in this cohort accessed a wide range of treatments and interventions. Five males and five females attended an ambulatory clinic associated with the service. One female attended a private psychiatrist in the community. Another woman received electroconvulsive therapy as an outpatient while living in an aged persons hostel. All 22 patients experienced positive symptoms such as auditory hallucinations, delusions, and ideas of reference. Ten men and 11 women received occupational therapy assessments. Figure 8.1 shows the range and frequency of occupational therapy interventions provided, demonstrating the complexity of need for this group. Four men and four women received neuropsychological assessment and

---

[1] Under the Mental Health Act 1986 (Victoria), Community Treatment Orders enable some involuntary patients to live in the community while they receive necessary treatment for their mental illness (Metropolitan Health and Aged Care Services Division, 2002b).

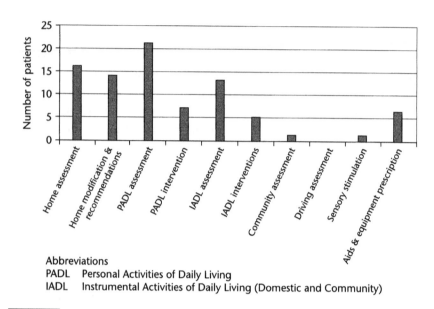

Abbreviations
PADL   Personal Activities of Daily Living
IADL   Instrumental Activities of Daily Living (Domestic and Community)

Figure 8.1 *Frequency of occupational therapy interventions.*

treatment, and of these, one woman received case management and behavioral interventions from the neuropsychologist as case manager over an extended period. Figure 8.2 documents the range and frequency of case management interventions provided by case managers to these people. Nine men and 12 women received specific social work interventions. Figure 8.3 documents the range and frequency of social work specific interventions provided to patients in the cohort.

Long-term psychotic illness has a significant impact on both family relationships and security of accommodation. Four men and three women had no family at all. A further two men and two women had tenuous links with one or two family members. Carers of two male and six female patients required referral to counselling agencies for problems associated with their caring role. For one man and five women, the involvement of the family member was at times an additional stressor. One woman was itinerant. One man and one woman were public housing tenants at the time of referral to the service. A further woman moved from derelict private rental to public housing. Two men lived in not-for-profit rooming houses (small room, communal cooking and bathroom facilities, no on-site care) and later moved to government-funded hostels providing all meals, domestic assistance, personal care prompting and assistance, and activity programs. Two men and two women had mutually

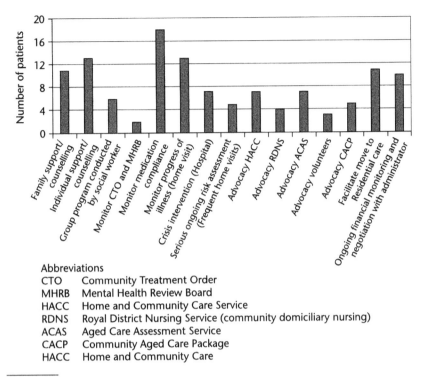

Abbreviations
CTO   Community Treatment Order
MHRB   Mental Health Review Board
HACC   Home and Community Care Service
RDNS   Royal District Nursing Service (community domiciliary nursing)
ACAS   Aged Care Assessment Service
CACP   Community Aged Care Package
HACC   Home and Community Care

Figure 8.2 *Frequency of case management interventions.*

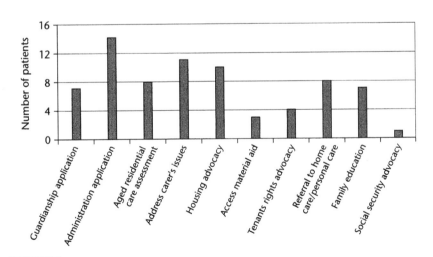

Figure 8.3 *Frequency of social work interventions.*

satisfactory family contact. Seven patients had at least one change of accommodation during their period of contact with our service. Four men and four women lived independently in their own homes alone. Two women each lived with a sibling. One man and two women lived in commercially owned supported residential services of very basic standard (shared rooms, communal bathrooms, meals and minimal personal assistance, no activity programs).

Similar to the experience of countries such as Canada and the United States (Minas, 1990, p.251), Australian society is rich in its cultural diversity. For this reason, standards for mental health services support the use of interpreters. While all 22 patients were capable of conversational English, 27.85% of the cohort (five men and one woman) had a first language other than English. The first languages other than English were Italian (two), German (one), Czechoslovakian (one), Greek (one), and Armenian (one). This is consistent with the first language profile of the local population of this age group. Interpreters were used for clinical interviews for five of these six individuals during clinical assessment and in relation to complex interventions. The other person declined the use of an interpreter.

Complex choices in therapeutic engagement

Therapeutic engagement with reluctant patients calls for creative activity by case managers and the multidisciplinary team. Many complex choices are encountered as team involvement with the patient unfolds.

Both at the beginning of an intervention and over time, how do we present our service in a way the patient perceives to be relevant and helpful? If the patient is concerned about possums[2] in the roof of their home, for example, then engagement may occur initially with a focus on that problem. How do we gain the trust of a patient or carer? Non-threatening visits or telephone calls, preferably at a regular and pre-arranged time, are often effective. When the patient or carer does open the door or answer the phone, how do we frame our communication to deal with the real issues in a helpful and acceptable way? When should the worker persist if the client declines an offer of assistance? When should family be contacted and what information should be provided to family within the constraints of the privacy legislation?

---

[2] Possums are Australian marsupials. Common urban species are about the size of a domestic cat.

In one case, the team became increasingly concerned about Gwen, a community patient in her mid-seventies receiving treatment under the Mental Health Act. Gwen has been diagnosed with early-onset schizophrenia and over the years has experienced a number of admissions to mental institutions (and latterly to the APMHS). There have been frequent appeals to the Mental Health Review Board because Gwen does not have insight into her illness and wishes to challenge her CTO. When unwell, Gwen also writes thought-disordered letters with paranoid themes to the manager of the service. These are responded to in accordance with the standard grievance procedures.

Gwen and her brother Bart live in the home of their childhood. This had become quite dilapidated and cluttered, and there were serious concerns about unsafe electrical wiring and the unusable bathroom and toilet. Although Gwen attended the required appointments for psychiatric review and for administering depot antipsychotic medication, she and Bart refused home visits.

The team encouraged the (social worker) case manager's initial outreach strategy of attempting to engage Gwen in a nonthreatening manner. Telephone calls remained unanswered, as were short letters. Cake or fruit were taken on home visits. If there was no answer, the small token was left at the door. In this way a degree of positive contact was maintained. Small gains were made, such as driving Gwen home after attending the (compulsory) clinic, assistance by a volunteer with her shopping, and Gwen's use of shower facilities at the APMHS. These were tasks that had practical meaning for Gwen. During this time she acknowledged that she was distressed over her home environment. Although she and Bart agreed to have their home assessed by the free Home Advisory Service, they declined to carry out the essential repairs identified by this service. Nor was the case manager able to enter into a discussion about alternative housing.

More recently, as a result of the case manager's ongoing monitoring, it was decided that Gwen required more assertive interventions and she was admitted to the acute aged psychiatry inpatient unit. This involuntary admission necessitated the involvement of police (as in the past) and was distressing for both Gwen and her brother, as well as for the team. As part of the hospital discharge plan, the occupational therapist assessed Gwen's home and clearly outlined the current risk to safety. In view of continued reluctance by Gwen and Bart to carry out repairs to their home, the social worker involved the Office of the Public Advocate to ensure that they had an alternative legal avenue for their interests.

While this action resulted in ensuring that safety issues were addressed, Gwen's view that such assertive intervention was an unnecessary intrusion compromised the original case manager's capacity to continue to work with her. Another member of the team has taken on that role. Gwen is showing signs of improved mental state and is happy to be able to use her bathroom again. It is expected that she will be a patient of the service until frail old age and possibly beyond. There will be other challenging risk issues for the case manager and the treating team to address. It is not expected that Gwen will welcome assertive outreach case management. The statutory appeals process and the APMHS grievance procedure are pathways available for her to express her view. Paradoxically, these pathways also provide a means of her keeping in touch with the services and a window into her mental state.

Complex choices in service delivery

Our experience shows that many patients with high care needs can eventually be integrated into community programs. Using existing community services available to the general population makes sense. Working with service providers can enhance their capacity to include patients with mental health problems. In this way we extend the movement towards integrating people with mental health problems into the general community. Service-specific programs can be a useful bridge for patients as they gain social skills and confidence. For some patients service-specific programs are essential for long periods. With adequate supports around a transition, many of our long-term vulnerable patients have been successfully integrated into community programs.

Community-based services are usually delivered by case managers, who may be psychiatric nurses, occupational therapists, social workers, psychologists, neuropsychologists, or psychiatrists. Dieticians, physiotherapists, podiatrists, music therapists, and speech therapists may contribute to client care as needed. There may be discipline-specific assessments and interventions, such as an occupational therapy personal care assessment using the Barthel index; site-specific interventions such as inpatient admission or the fitting of aids and equipment to the home; or alternative interventions such as the introduction of the patient to a community-based social support program. If necessary, a center-based rehabilitation group program can be provided by the APMHS. In a well-integrated team, discipline-specific interventions are not always delivered by the professional who developed them. For example, there may be reasons of therapeutic engagement, gender, language or culture which suggest that the female Italian-speaking case manager, qualified in social work, delivers home aids selected by the occupational therapist on the team. Team members from various disciplines may be involved in the application of a behavior management strategy developed by the neuropsychologist after complex assessment and planning. Not surprisingly, patients wish to know about the qualifications as well as the role of their case manager. This information should usually be volunteered by the case manager and should always be stated if asked.

Services from the wider community, such as home help or personal care, may be used to support the patient at home. Some advocacy may be required by the case manager to secure an appropriate level of service. The patient may be physically able, but require prompting and the structure of regular visits initiated by a personal carer to keep up an adequate level of personal and domestic hygiene. There may be a need to explain the extent of the disability to Home and Community Care (HACC) service providers more accustomed to providing care and assistance to patients with obvious physical disabilities. A proactive APMHS will offer in-service training and ongoing liaison to personal care workers and home care workers from the relevant agencies, to ensure that workers and managers are confident and well informed when assisting patients with a mental illness. This also offers the opportunity for de-stigmatization of the patient and mental illness in general.

In our experience, it is possible to develop a working relationship with community house programs and social support programs to integrate selected patients into courses and activities that are of genuine interest to them. English and mathematics classes at a learning exchange or a local patchwork circle provide a welcoming and encouraging link for patients with the wider community. In the short term, however, and sometimes in the long term, some patients are unable to move confidently into such an environment. Rehabilitation group programs are conducted by the APMHS, with the goal of such patients 'graduating' to groups in the wider community while still receiving case management for mental health issues from the APMHS. These rehabilitation groups offer recognition and appreciation of the patient as an interesting and worthwhile person, validation of the patient's experience of mental illness, and the opportunity to develop social and practical skills to strengthen their capacity to function independently in the community. There have been many successful outcomes for patients attending groups conducted on this model. Groups are, of course, not for everyone. Case management with an individual service plan developed in consultation with the patient and, where possible, with significant family members, can provide holistic support and monitoring of the person's mental state and general well-being. Mental health advocacy groups can also provide beneficial mutual assistance as well as addressing systemic problems regarding services and community attitudes.

Josef, diagnosed with late-onset paranoid schizophrenia, provides an example of someone for whom ongoing support from the multidisciplinary team and participation in the APMHS rehabilitation group program led to significant improvements in his situation. Now in his late seventies, Josef emigrated from Eastern Europe after World War II and has no family in Australia. He worked in construction until retirement, lived in boarding houses, never married, and remained socially isolated. When he was first admitted into the APMHS, his diet was limited and his room was poorly kept. Neuropsychological testing revealed no cognitive deficit. Josef has a good command of English, yet rarely communicated beyond indicating 'yes' or 'no'. Although there was an improvement to his mental state with the introduction of depot antipsychotic medication, Josef remained isolative and guarded, with poor insight. He indicated that he suffered nightmares about his traumatic war experiences, but revealed few other details about his life or interests. Discharge planning from hospital included allocation of a case manager to monitor symptomatology as well as his broader physical and emotional well-being.

In an attempt to reduce his social isolation and assist him to regain social and functional skills, Josef was introduced to the APMHS rehabilitation group program. He was encouraged to attend weekly group sessions facilitated by the social worker and the occupational therapist. The group consisted of six men with a similar diagnosis at different stages of rehabilitation. Members participated in discussions, group activities, and nutritious afternoon tea. For clients with negative symptoms, lack of motivation for activities of daily living is difficult to overcome. A supportive environment is needed for practicing social skills and building relationships. The men were encouraged to be sensitive and tolerant to other group participants' views (and behaviors). They were also encouraged to greet and farewell one another politely.

During the first few months, Josef was encouraged to establish a routine by arriving to the group on time. Communication continued to be minimal but he appeared content to follow direction from the facilitator of the group. Over the following year, trust and rapport were established to the point where the case manager and group facilitator were able to work with him to achieve placement in residential care. This proved to be a significant factor in improving his overall health. Josef's personal care improved, his home environment was now clean and he enjoyed having regular meals. Supervision was provided with medication, which allowed for the depot antipsychotic to be ceased and oral medication commenced, minimizing risk of side effects. Signs of enthusiasm became apparent during group work. This continued to expand when the group as a whole chose to participate in the hospital-wide 'football tipping'[3] competition. As time went on, Josef spoke about his interest in football and his achievements in this sport as a young man. This was the most he had communicated since his admission to hospital. Josef was now an established and contributing member of the group. To the group's delight, they won the competition and celebrated this achievement with awards presented by the Director of Aged Psychiatry – an event covered on the local evening television news.

Josef continues to have a tendency to remain isolative and communicates minimally, but he is much more readily engaged in meaningful activities and is able to express pleasure in his achievements. He has recently agreed to join an alternative group in the general community, which provides a long-term structured diversional focus. The practice of integrating long-term clients into programs in the general community may present additional challenges to clients who are initially reluctant to engage with the service. It is therefore important that this is done in a sensitive and supportive manner. The multidisciplinary team should avoid the risk of our expectations for clients remaining too low. Re-referral pathways should be clear and accessible to the client and to the wider service system.

Decision making for the manager and team

How do we ensure that the patient receives the benefit of having a consistent case manager, while receiving the full range of skills available from all members of the multidisciplinary team? Workers benefit from maintaining their discipline-specific skills while applying their additionally acquired case management skills. Discipline-specific supervision and staff development programs are essential to maintain and enhance this aspect of the worker's team contribution. Research activities from both team- and discipline-specific perspectives are essential to strengthen the knowledge base of work in this field.

---

[3] A popular form of forecasting weekly results of the major winter sport in Melbourne, involving a token payment and shared rewards for successful participants.

Where a worker provides a discipline-specific skill in person, he or she may be introduced to the patient by the case manager, who explains the role of this other team member. The discipline-specific worker may then visit alone when the patient is confident for this to occur. There may be a change to a case manager of a different discipline when a patient's circumstances change or staff move on.

How can the team work most effectively? Experienced leadership enables team members to function confidently as differing opinions are expressed in team meetings and while carrying out care plans. Robust creative brainstorming in team meetings provides good quality assurance and monitoring of risk factors, and addresses accountability issues in a holistic way. The multidisciplinary team can use varied perspectives to develop innovative strategies, minimizing the restrictiveness of the interventions. Team dynamics should be conducive to clear, honest nonhierarchical discussion, respectful of the contributions of each member of the team. Long-term case managers may well have a stronger estimation of the client's strengths and vulnerabilities than is held by other members of the team. Case managers benefit from the team's confidence in their in-depth understanding of the client's capacity to change. The resulting decisions and plans should be clearly documented and understood by all team members involved in applying the strategies. Where possible, the needs of family members should also be considered in the care plan. Family members can often alert the case manager when signs of a relapse are noted, as they may be aware of symptomatology that is individualized to the patient.

Supervision from the team leader as well as discipline-specific supervision will optimize the contributions from team members to the work of the service. Geographic co-location of the various components of the service facilitates a high quality of formal and informal communication and interdisciplinary understanding, thus enhancing team performance.

Conclusion

The multidisciplinary team has scope for a wide range of resources to assist patients of a mental health service for older people. Long-term involvement enables a refinement of the treatment approach beyond acute clinical interventions, with a detailed consideration of the patients' individual needs and circumstances. More subtle improvements such as a patient's capacity to contain emotional responses or to express feelings in a more socially appropriate way can be supported through long-term involvement. Long-term contact also enables changes such as a move to more appropriate accommodation, with the improved physical environment in turn leading to health benefits. Many long-term patients will have a longer history with the agency than their case manager does. Regular and consistent documentation in the file will contribute to continuity of care for individuals as case managers change and staff move on. Team-specific and discipline-specific supervision, and a physical working environment that promotes formal and informal communication, enhance team performance. Close links with social services and social support programs in the community promote community integration for patients. For workers, there is considerable satisfaction to be derived from working with patients for long enough to see improvements in their patient's well-being and overall social functioning.

Multidisciplinary community-based long-term case management, with additional rehabilitative group work as appropriate, has demonstrated long-term benefits for clients of our service. Well-designed research into this mode of service would strengthen our work through evidence-based practice. A multidisciplinary approach applies more broadly as well: Palmer et al (1999) have argued that to help improve outcomes for older people with schizophrenia there is a need for the establishment of interdisciplinary collaboration among researchers, clinicians, government and industry representatives, and advocacy groups. As Palmer et al have also indicated, patients who survive into old age with schizophrenia may themselves teach us about skills for coping with the challenges of the illness.

References

Commonwealth of Australia, *National Mental Health Strategy: National Standards for Mental Health Services*, endorsed by Australian Health Ministers Advisory Council, National Mental Health Working Group (Australian Government Publishing Service: Canberra, 1996).

Kilian R, Lindenbach I, Löbig U et al, Self-perceived social integration and the use of day centers of persons with severe and persistent schizophrenia living in the community: a qualitative analysis, *Soc Psychiatry Psychiatr Epidemiol* (2001) 36:545–52.

Metropolitan Health and Aged Care Services Division, *Victoria's Mental Health Services Consumer Guide: How Case Management Can Help You* (Victorian Department of Human Services: Melbourne, Victoria, 2002a).

Metropolitan Health and Aged Care Services Division, *Community Treatment Order and Restricted Community Treatment Order: About Your Rights* (Victorian Department of Human Services: Melbourne, Victoria, 2002b).

Minas IH, Mental health in a culturally diverse society. In: Reid J, Trompf P, eds, *The Health of Immigrant Australia* (Harcourt Grace Jovanovich: Sydney, 1990) 250–87.

Mohamed S, Kaschow JW, Granholm E, Jeste DV, Community-based treatment of schizophrenia and other severe mental illnesses. In: Cohen CI, ed, *Schizophrenia in Later Life* (American Psychiatric Association: Washington, DC, 2003) 205–22.

Palmer BW, Heaton SC, Jeste DV, Older patients with schizophrenia: challenges in the coming decades, *Psychiatr Serv* (1999) 50:1178–83.

Raschko R, Late-life mental illness outreach and in-home interventions, *Journal of the California Alliance for the Mentally Ill* (1998) 9:60–2.

Shaw WS, Patterson TL, Semple SJ et al, Use of community support services by middle-aged and older patients with psychotic disorders, *Psychiatr Serv* (2000) 51:506–12.

Spaid WM, Giving and receiving social supports for elderly mentally ill people, *J Case Manag* (1998) 7:24–30.

chapter 9

Residential care for the elderly with early- or late-onset schizophrenia

Christine McDougall and Heather Rota

Introduction

The late twentieth century saw a shift in the provision of long-term care for persons with chronic psychiatric illnesses away from large stand-alone psychiatric institutions to smaller community-based facilities. As part of this process, many older people with schizophrenia have been relocated from long-stay 'back wards' to a mixture of community-based residential services.

In general, people with late-onset schizophrenia (late paraphrenia) are more likely to be treated in the domain of the acute inpatient and community service arms of an aged psychiatry service, with only approximately 10% of them presenting for long-term residential care (Hassett, personal communication). The rest of the current cohort of old people with schizophrenia are more likely to be 'graduates' of the previous mental health system. The term graduates was introduced by Arie and Jolley (1982) for people described as 'Patients who entered hospitals for the mentally ill before modern methods of treatment were available and have grown old in them after many years there'. With the change sweeping through most developed countries in the latter decades of the twentieth century, resulting in closure of large institutions, the term must now also be considered to apply to those elderly people with long-term histories of mental illness who live in the community and require ongoing support and management. There is very little in the literature addressing the care needs of this group of people in residential (nursing home) care. As this group of patients succumb to the physical disabilities of the aging process they will increasingly require nursing home level of care, that is, care that in the past had been provided in large mental health institutions.

Throughout the world aged psychiatry services are facing the challenge of where and how to house and care for these elderly patients with special needs. The state of Victoria in Australia is unique in having a comprehensive aged psychiatry service system, supported through policy and funding by the Health Department of the state government. A component of this system is the provision of specifically designed, purpose-built and -staffed aged psychiatry nursing homes. There are 17 of these homes throughout the state and all are linked to a comprehensive aged psychiatry service and form an integral part of these services. These homes also receive significant funding from the federal government under the same scheme that funds all other aged care residential homes in Australia. Principles that underpin care in Victorian aged psychiatry nursing homes can be extrapolated for use in areas under other systems of management.

This chapter examines how the management of the graduates, and the smaller number of late-onset patients, can be achieved in residential care settings that are noninstitutional in nature, design, and philosophy. In most developed countries, nurses in residential care settings provide leadership in the management of older residents. The humanism that underpins nursing values and the emphasis placed by nurses on autonomy, personal dignity, health promotion, and disease prevention are particularly relevant to the unique psychosocial needs of older persons with schizophrenia in these settings. The disciplines of social work (Brody, 1977), psychiatry (Bienenfeld and Wheeler, 1989; Grossberg et al, 1990), psychology (Smyer et al, 1992), and nursing (Taube et al, 1984; Santmyer and Roca, 1991) all have proposed models for delivering better psychosocial care in the nursing home setting. What is common to all of these proposed models is the use of psychiatrically trained professionals, using appropriate assessment tools to ensure the most appropriate care and treatment for the elderly psychiatric patient.

One of the primary areas for concern in regard to the aged with psychiatric disabilities who have moved from an institution to a more relaxed home-like environment is the relative freedom that they now encounter. For a small number of these relocated persons fear of the unknown can lead to an exacerbation of behaviors that may have been unnoticed or unremarked in the institution. Studies of elderly people moved from institutional care to community units (Meehan et al, 2001) have shown that after an initial resettling period the patients did not exhibit long-term functioning or behavioral deficits, although others (Farhall et al, 1996) found that there was an increase in agitation and aggression following relocation. Other patients will have behaviors that are challenging and will continue to be so irrespective of the environment. There is also the challenge of cognitive impairment that is the 'double jeopardy' of schizophrenia.

Neuropsychological changes are evident early in the course of the illness, and then in later life a number of factors contribute to further decline in cognitive functioning. The deficits are not as severe or as disabling as those found in dementias but they can be more difficult to deal with than the positive symptoms of the illness.

The staff

This shift in the focus of care has caused, and continues to cause, substantial anxiety among nonspecialist staff. Specific training and introduction of systems and services to assist in caring for this cohort of patients would be the most appropriate approach to minimize this anxiety, and to improve the quality of care for the elderly with schizophrenia. One of the most important things for nursing staff to remember is the concept of self and an awareness of the personhood of the patients/residents. Personhood 'is a standing or status that is bestowed upon one human being, by others, in the context of relationship and social beings. It implies recognition, respect and trust' (Kitwood, 1997). This should be one of the driving philosophies behind all of the work that is done so that it becomes ingrained in the work culture consciousness.

It is not true to say that if you are a health professional you do not have stereotyped ageist views that can be common among a group. The ageist attitudes of some health professionals do inhibit their ability to provide holistic care to the patient. This can lead to a workforce culture whereby patients are dehumanized and starved of psychological acknowledgment and care. Where such attitudes are identified, it is the responsibility of the service to acknowledge the deficit and to set about creating a set of strategies based on service structure, orientation, education, performance management, and quality assurance by which the values and expectations of the service are reflected in the work design and practice to promote quality professional practice and positive aging attitudes.

Working with the staff

In-services, staff consultation, and case conferences provide experiential, case-related information to improve staff understanding and provide examples of management approaches from which the individual residents or the group of residents can benefit.

Allowing the staff of the nursing homes to appreciate the patients/residents as people rather than 'problems', can often be achieved by use of life histories and discussions with families and significant others. This introduces the staff to a person who they no longer see as egocentric, with demanding behaviors, but rather as a person who has developed particular coping strategies over a lifetime, which has often been a very difficult and challenged life. Presentations of life histories can occur in training sessions, or nursing staff handover time, or can be maintained in easily accessible places for staff to read in quiet moments during the day. It is important to allow time for discussion and reflection on how these life histories may impact on the behaviors presenting in later life. During discussion about a particular elderly person with schizophrenia, staff should be encouraged to talk about how they feel when confronted by particular behaviors and also to imagine how the patient/resident themselves may be experiencing the same situation. Common sources of frustration and stress for staff are when people display anger or persistent repetitive, apparently meaningless, behaviors or are generally demanding in their behaviors. Evaluation of medical issues, medication and biological aspects should also be explored, which then enables staff to expand their knowledge base and to be involved in the complete management of the resident/patient. By addressing care-related problems and solutions, the staff become a very powerful peer group and can become more open to dealing with conceptual issues.

Medical care

The primary medical care of patients is the responsibility of the general practitioner (GP). Many GPs do not have extensive knowledge of schizophrenia and particularly the presentation of the illness in the elderly. Ensuring that the nursing staff and other care staff have significant knowledge and understanding of the issues and the individuals under their care can only enhance the provision of care that the GP can provide, particularly when called upon to prescribe psychotropic medication.

Direct medical care of the patient by the GP is one of the major strengths of the aged psychiatry nursing homes and is integral to the policy of allowing the elderly with schizophrenia to have access to the same level of care as their peers who do not have a mental illness. However, as also stated previously, not all GPs have an understanding of the special needs of this group of elderly people. The consultant old age psychiatrist is the ideal person to provide a consultative service to the nursing homes and the GPs. This is done according to local policy in each nursing home across the state, where it may be that a senior registrar in old age psychiatry will provide the regular visits and receive supervision from a consultant. Ideally the consultant psychiatrist, or senior registrar, makes regular visits and meets with staff for case discussions. According to the needs of the particular nursing home, visits can be arranged with all patients being reviewed on a regular rotating six-month basis, with additional reviews performed on an 'as required basis'. Some GPs prefer to conduct a 'round' of their patients with the psychiatrist, thereby taking the opportunity to discuss management and drug therapy directly with the specialist. Educational breakfasts, with either the consultant or an academic psychiatrist, and the GPs have proved popular at the nursing homes in our service, and provide the GPs with an opportunity to discuss wider issues with relation to aged psychiatry, as well as individual patients. The psychiatrist is also an important resource for the nursing staff and education sessions can be organized for staff to attend with the specialist. Not only does this provide the staff with valuable information, it provides them with an opportunity to ask questions and discuss individual situations and validates their role as valuable members of the team.

Assessments

Initially patients/residents need to undergo comprehensive assessments. Mental status and cognitive assessments would, ideally, have been completed prior to admission to the nursing home. These assessments are most usually conducted in the relevant inpatient assessment unit of the aged psychiatry service. If this is not the case they can be completed once the person has been admitted. It is unusual in Victoria for any person to be admitted to a psychogeriatric nursing home without first having an admission to an assessment unit. The further assessments completed by the nursing staff should be designed and proven to be of value as an information tool that will assist in developing care and management plans for the resident. The tools used must be reliable, validated, and have meaning. Individual assessments and skill development improve overall functioning, well-being, and quality of life for the residents. It is important that the family or carers are invited to be involved in all aspects of the assessment and care planning of the resident.

The following assessments need to be completed to give a clear picture to the staff of how to manage the resident:

- Communication
- Mobility
- Nutrition/hydration
- Hygiene, dressing, grooming
- Toileting
- Activities of daily living
- Social needs
- Medication
- Psychotic symptomatology (hallucinations, delusions)
- Podiatry
- Dietary needs
- Wandering/intrusive behavior
- Physically aggressive behavior
- Damage to self or others
- Emotional dependence
- Family needs
- Verbally aggressive behavior.

While some of the above may not seem to specifically relate to psychiatric illness, the nurse needs an awareness of the entire person and all things that can affect them and their behavior. The need for physical assessment is paramount for a number of reasons:

1. Co-morbid conditions may adversely affect the clinical course of treatment of schizophrenia.
2. Persons with schizophrenia may under-report symptoms because the disorder may increase pain tolerance.
3. Deficits in cognitive processes may diminish the patient's insight about medical as well as psychiatric illness.
4. Neuroleptic treatment may reduce pain sensitivity (Cohen et al, 2000).

Care plans and management plans need to be individualized according to the result of the assessments and tailored to the individual needs of the residents. The tasks for the nurses to consider here are the usefulness of the information they have gathered and the transformation of this into a meaningful management plan. Individualized coping strategies and behaviors of the patient need to be considered in the formulation of these plans, while keeping in mind the requirements of regulating and funding bodies.

People with schizophrenia are not a homogenous group and are likely to present with many and varied behaviors and symptoms.

Medication

There are no prescriptions for the care of these people that can be universally applied; only principles of care. Medication should not be seen as a first resort but rather an adjunct to the care that is provided. An unpublished study conducted by one of the authors (Rota), in the nursing home she manages, showed a 50% reduction in the use of psychotropic medication following assessments and introduction of alternate strategies for managing behaviors. Comprehensive assessment, staff training and staff brainstorming sessions, behavioral charting and auditing of intervention strategies achieved this. Consultations with the GPs and psychiatrists about medications and presenting problems were also invaluable in this process.

Environment

Environment is a key factor in the management of people with behavioral problems. The rigid structure of institutional care provides safety for them and being given more choice and opportunity for individual expression can in itself be a challenge. Newer homes for the aged person are designed with more of a sense of freedom and individuality. While this is a good thing, it can be difficult for people, on initially relocating, who are used to a more structured environment. Rituals and routines that provide comfort and security should be allowed to continue as much as possible, as long as they do not impinge on the rights of the other residents. Over time it is possible to work individually with people to allow them to adjust to greater freedoms.

Freedom of movement, light, use of color and textures are very important. Too often in residential settings a television is used as a 'baby sitter'. In our homes we have a television in a smaller sitting room away from the larger room and residents can also have one in their room if desired. Music can be used therapeutically at different times of the day and also used in individual sessions with residents, catering to their tastes and moods at the time.

Other strategies that have been found to be effective are aromatherapy, pet therapy, dance therapy, art, walking, taking people to places of interest, and remembrance from their past. Some activities can be organized for a group or at times for an individual. It is important to remember that goals we hope to achieve with the patient may not be attained at the first attempt.

Conclusion and future directions

As the trend towards de-institutionalization continues and more and more people with schizophrenia age in the community, the need to care for them in aged care residential homes is going to increase. A large number of these future users of the residential homes are not going to come from a background of institutional care, rather they are going to come from the community where they have been supported by the adult health system. They will have far more idiosyncratic ways of managing their life and illness than the graduates we now care for. There is a need for training and development now and also to prepare for the future for the new 'graduates' who are going to use the residential aged care homes. Exciting and challenging times lie ahead for mental health planners when looking to provision of care for the elderly with schizophrenia.

References

Arie T, Jolley DJ, Making services work: organisation and style of psychogeriatric services. In: Levy R, Post F, eds, *The Psychiatry of Late Life* (Blackwell: Oxford, 1982) 222–51.

Bienenfeld F, Wheeler BG, Psychiatric services to nursing homes: a liaison model, *Hosp Community Psychiatry* (1989) **40**:793–4.

Brody EM, *Long Term Care of Older People: A Practical Guide* (Human Sciences: New York, 1977).

Cohen C, Cohen G, Blank K et al, Schizophrenia and older adults, an overview: directions for research and policy, *Am J Geriatric Psychiatry* (2000) **8**:19–28.

Farhall J, Trower T, Attwood R et al, Evaluating the short term impact of moving from psychiatric hospital to community care unit. Proceedings of the *6th Mental Health Services Conference*, Brisbane, Australia (1996).

Grossberg GT, Rakhghanda H, Szwabo PA et al, Psychiatric problems in the nursing homes, *J Am Geriatr Soc* (1990) **38**:907–17.

Kitwood T, *Dementia Reconsidered* (Open University Press: London, 1997).

Meehan T, Robertson S, Vermeer C, The impact of relocation on elderly patients with mental illness, *Aust N Z J Ment Health Nurs* (2001) **10**:236.

Santmyer KS, Roca RP, Geropsychiatry in long term care: a nurse centred approach, *J Am Geriatr Soc* (1991) **39**:156–9.

Smyer MA, Brannon D, Cohen M, Improving nursing care through training and job design, *Gerontologist* (1992) **32**:327–33.

Taube A, Burns BJ, Kessler L, Patients of psychiatrists and psychologists in office-practice 1980, *Am Psychol* (1984) **39**:1435–47.

chapter 10

De-stigmatization of elderly people with early- or late-onset schizophrenia

James Lindesay

Introduction

People with mental disorders have to contend not only with their illness, but also with the fear and disapproval it provokes in others. This stigma adds considerably to the burden of mental illness, and it is the duty of health professionals to challenge and prevent it wherever possible. This is easier said than done. With few exceptions, psychiatric stigma is widespread and deep-rooted in both developed and developing societies, and addressing it effectively requires effort and action at many levels, from the individual to the international. At the level of organizations such as the United Nations and the World Health Organization (WHO), the message is clear: 'All persons with a mental disorder (or who are being treated as such persons) shall be treated humanely and with respect for the inherent dignity of the human person' (United Nations, 1991). The challenge is to translate these ideals into reality, a task in which health professionals working with mentally ill people have an important role to play.

This chapter outlines how we can help to reduce the stigma associated with psychosis in old age. To date, most of the discussion of and research into psychiatric stigma has been in younger adults, particularly those with schizophrenia and other psychotic disorders. While much of this is also relevant to the elderly population, there is also a need to address the 'double jeopardy' of both psychiatric stigma and the stigma against old age. This chapter will discuss briefly the causes of these stigmatizing attitudes, and then examine how they might be challenged and their effects mitigated. This subject was addressed recently in a Technical Consensus Statement, published jointly by WHO and the World Psychiatric Association (WPA) (WHO/WPA, 2002; Graham et al, 2003).

Causes of stigma

In order to address psychiatric stigma, it is necessary to have some under-standing of why it arises, so that an effective counter-strategy can be developed. Stigma is a process whereby certain individuals or groups within society are marked out and devalued. Although it is a universal social phenomenon, its origins and purposes remain unclear. It arises out of the cognitive processes that evaluate threat and risk, organize social knowledge, and determine self-perception (Hilton and von Hippel, 1996; Crocker et al, 1998), and appears to be a means by which human groups alert themselves to potential physical and economic danger from among their number (Buss, 1999). The roots of psychiatric stigma lie primarily in the perceived dangerousness of individuals with mental illness (especially schizophrenia); they are seen as unpredictable, unmanageable, and untreatable. There is also an economic driver, in that mental illness is regarded as being under the control of the affected individuals, who are therefore not 'pulling their weight' within their communities. Elderly people with mental disorders may be perceived as less dangerous, and so be less stigmatized on these grounds; however, this is probably more than compensated for by the perception of economic burden that they are thought to represent. In some cultures, eccentric and isolated elderly people can attract very damaging and dangerous labels, such as 'witch' and 'pedophile'.

These stigmatizing stereotypes, born of ignorance and fear, lead to prejudicial attitudes, which in turn lead to discrimination against the stigmatized group. This discrimination operates at the levels of both individual behavior and social policy, and is manifest in various forms of reducing or nullifying mentally ill people's equal enjoyment of their rights, through acts of avoidance, withholding help, coercion, and segregation (Corrigan and Watson, 2002). The stigmatized group is thereby marginalized, the negative stereotype is reinforced, and the vicious circle is completed.

Action against stigma

The challenge facing anti-stigma strategies and campaigns is how to break this vicious circle of stigma, prejudice, and discrimination. Addressing stigma and prejudice requires action to change beliefs and attitudes, while addressing discrimination is more a matter of changing the legal and policy frameworks in which discriminatory decisions are made (WHO/WPA, 2002). Three broad strategic approaches to reducing public stigma have been described, and to some extent researched: protest, education, and contact (Corrigan and Watson, 2002). Protest strategies may be effective in reducing media misrepresentations of mental illness, and can be important in campaigns to challenge discrimination in law and social policy. However, as current controversies about 'political correctness' demonstrate, protest can also have the opposite effect of reinforcing stigmatizing attitudes in some social groups. It may be more effective when related to specific cases rather than general issues ('human interest'), and when combined with education and contact. This approach underlies the 'advocacy' model of patient support and empowerment.

Regarding education and contact, there is some evidence that psychiatric stigma can be reduced by providing people with information about mental illness (Penn et al, 1994; Corrigan and Penn, 1999; Holmes et al, 1999), and by increasing their contact with mentally ill individuals (Kolodziej and Johnson, 1996). However, the effect of these interventions does not appear to be very large or long-lasting (Morrison et al, 1979; Keane, 1991; Wolff et al, 1996). People learn to give appropriate responses to post-intervention surveys, but this may not reflect a change in attitudes or behavior (Haghighat, 2001). Unfortunately, the current evidence base for these approaches is limited by the fact that most of the studies are small, laboratory-based, short-term, and focused on individuals. We need large-scale, long-term naturalistic evaluations that examine change at the level of the individual and the social and institutional structures, if we are to identify those strategies that make meaningful differences to patients' lives.

Broad educational strategies are expensive, and may not work. Smaller-scale interventions may be more effective, particularly if they target those groups with whom elderly patients have most day-to-day contact, such as their families, health professionals, and other carers. It is unfortunately the case that psychiatric stigma is still widespread in health and social services, in all professions and in all specialties, including psychiatry. This has serious consequences for mentally ill patients; not only do they receive poorer quality treatment and care (e.g. Folsom et al, 2002), they are less likely to co-operate with what is offered. Patients with schizophrenia perceive health professionals as either helpful or unhelpful, depending on how they judge the health professional perceives them (Brammer, 2001), and it is likely that 'unhelpful' health professionals will have less success with these patients than 'helpful' ones. All health professionals need to examine their own attitudes and practice to ensure that they are free from stigma and discrimination. An educational approach emphasizing the impact of their attitudes on patient outcomes may be helpful in achieving this.

Health professionals also have an important role in any campaign against psychiatric stigma, and the WHO/WPA Technical Consensus Statement lists the many ways in which they can contribute (Box 10.1). Most importantly, they are in a position to encourage the development of better, more acceptable services and more effective treatments. As the examples of epilepsy and AIDS in the developed world demonstrate, improvements in services and treatments are probably the most effective means of changing attitudes towards a stigmatized disorder.

Another group on whom stigma-reducing educational strategies can and should be focused is the patient's family. In the case of elderly people, this will usually involve their spouses, siblings, and children, if any. These individuals are likely to be the group with whom the patient has most contact, and whose opinions and respect they most value. As well as information about the mental illness, families also need to be reassured about any risk that the patient may present to themselves or others, and it is important to address any anxieties they may have about heritability. It should be borne in mind that psychiatric stigma often extends to the patient's family, and may have adverse consequences for their own mental health (Ostman and Kjellin, 2002). In some cultures, shame and stigma may result in total exclusion of the patient from society. In younger adults, there are positive reports of a sibling support program in Canada, which involves family members in planning to provide a stable future for their schizophrenic relatives (Thompson, 2003). It is not known if a similar approach would work with elderly patients.

It must not be forgotten that, as members of their society, people with mental illness are likely to share its common attitudes and beliefs, including those about mental illness. Less is known about self-stigma than about public stigma, but there is evidence from focus groups and personal accounts that testifies to the severe adverse impact that it has on self-esteem, particularly

Box 10.1 Roles, responsibilities and opportunities for stigma reduction

Health professionals (including paid care workers) should:

- Ensure that their own practice is free from stigma and discrimination
- Join with government, nongovernmental organizations (NGOs) and patients and carers to plan and develop services, and ensure that they avoid stigma and discrimination
- Ensure that all educational and continuing professional development curricula contain:
  - Appropriate material on mental disorders in old age
  - Training to develop awareness of stigma and discrimination
  - Training to ensure that assessments and planned care provision take positive account of aspects of mental health and aging
  - Continuous supervision (coaching)
- Ensure that due weight is given to issues of mental disorders in old age in the professional research agenda
- Ensure that professional bodies have policies in place to identify and reduce stigma and discrimination
- Ensure that local workplace policies are in place to identify and reduce stigma and discrimination
- Provide information and advice to individual patients, carers and families regarding:
  - Disorders
  - Treatments
  - Local community specialist services
  - The work of relevant NGOs
- Help patients, families and other professional carers to cope with the stigma and discrimination that they experience
- Provide accurate information to journalists and the media
- Disseminate good evidence-based practice to ensure early identification and effective treatment of mental disorders in older people
- Assure and regulate the competence of care providers

Source: WHO/WPA (2002)

when compounded by the effects of public stigma (Gallo, 1994; Wright et al, 2000). Ironically, effective treatment of psychosis that restores insight may make the patient more vulnerable to self-stigma. It is not known whether or not older people with disorders such as schizophrenia are more self-stigmatizing. On the one hand, they may be more likely to share the more stigmatizing attitudes of their generation (Stuart and Arboleda-Florez, 2001);

on the other, an illness appearing late in life may have less impact on a more securely established sense of self-esteem than one with its onset in early adulthood. Indeed, it is likely that those whose onset of illness was in early adulthood will be severely affected by a lifetime of discrimination and rejection. Addressing self-stigma involves action to restore self-respect and self-efficacy, for example through participation in activities leading to the acquisition of new skills, or in educational programs aimed at challenging stigma.

Another approach to reducing psychiatric stigma involves focusing on what it is that makes the patient's mental illness *visible* to others, notably behavior, abnormal movements associated with drug treatment, and association with specific stigmatized services (Davidson, 2002). To some extent, this approach runs counter to the philosophy of stigma reduction through education and contact, but it has the potential advantage that it involves actions and strategies that fall within the scope of the individual patient and practitioner. Stigmatizing behaviors in schizophrenia include those related to psychotic symptoms (e.g. responding to hallucinations or acting on delusions), those related to the negative symptoms (e.g. self-neglect), and poor social skills (Penn et al, 2000). These may be reduced by intervention strategies such as cognitive behavior therapy, social skills training, and the development and retention of effective self-care skills, although evidence for their effectiveness in elderly patients is largely lacking. There is also no evidence that these interventions lead to a reduction in the stigma and discrimination experienced by patients. Incidentally, changes in public standards of behavior may also lead to changes in what is and is not regarded as indicative of mental illness. For example, it is interesting to note that talking to yourself in public has become much less stigmatizing thanks to the widespread use of mobile phones, particularly the hands-free variety.

There are plenty of reasons, including stigma reduction, why drug treatment should always aim to minimize the risk of the patient developing disabling side-effects. The newer atypical antipsychotic drugs are now the treatment of choice for schizophrenia and other psychoses developing in old age (see Chapter 6). Elderly patients whose schizophrenia started early in adult life are likely to have had long exposures to conventional antipsychotic drugs, and to suffer from significant intractable movement disorders as a result. However, there may be some benefit to be gained from transferring them to an atypical antipsychotic drug (see Chapter 6).

The third visible stigma identified by Davidson (2002) is the patients' association with stigmatized services and institutions. He advocates providing as much care as possible in alternative settings, such as geriatric wards in the case of elderly patients with a mental illness. There are probably limits to the extent to which this is practically achievable, particularly if the patient is acutely ill, and this approach risks the patient becoming highly stigmatized by others within the alternative environment (clients and staff). However, there is certainly scope for the greater use of a wider range of supportive settings for patients in the recovery and remission phases of their illness. It is also the case that if psychiatric treatment and care is provided in well-designed, attractive settings, it will be more acceptable and less stigmatizing.

While some approaches to reduce the public visibility of mental illness may be helpful, others may do more harm than good; one study found that keeping the history of psychiatric treatment a secret or avoiding situations where rejection might occur had no effect on employability or on levels of patients' distress and demoralization (Link et al, 1991). The avoidance strategy in fact made matters significantly worse. This study also looked at the effect of educating others about their situation, and this had no effect either. The authors make the point that stigma is a 'social problem' and not an 'individual trouble', and that its effects are not easily overcome by individual coping strategies.

Conclusions

Elderly people with schizophrenia are no less vulnerable than younger adults to the adverse effects of stigma and discrimination. The extent to which these effects can be prevented or mitigated is uncertain, but health professionals have a responsibility to help and to lead, not only in their daily practice with patients, but also as service developers, managers, educators, and researchers. As the WHO/WPA Technical Consensus Statement concludes: 'The development of effective, well-regarded health and social support services for older people with mental disorders should be the first priority of any strategy to reduce stigma and discrimination' (WHO/WPA, 2002).

References

Brammer SV, How persons with schizophrenia experience connecting with mental health professionals, *Dissertation Abstracts International: Section B (Sciences and Engineering)* (2001) **61**:3504.

Buss D, *Evolutionary Psychology* (Allyn and Bacon: Boston, 1999).

Corrigan PW, Penn DL, Lessons from social psychology on discrediting psychiatric stigma, *Am Psychol* (1999) **54**:765–6.

Corrigan PW, Watson AC, Understanding the impact of stigma on people with mental illness, *World Psychiatry* (2002) **1**:16–19.

Crocker J, Major B, Steele C, Social stigma. In: Gilbert D, Fiske ST, Lindzey G, eds, *The Handbook of Social Psychology*, Vol. 2 (McGraw-Hill: New York, 1998).

Davidson M, What else can we do to combat stigma?, *World Psychiatry* (2002) **1**:22–3.

Folsom DP, McCahill M, Bartels SJ et al, Medical comorbidity and receipt of medical care by older homeless people with schizophrenia or depression, *Psychiatr Serv* (2002) **53**:1456–60.

Gallo KM, First person account: self-stigmatization, *Schizophr Bull* (1994) **20**:407–10.

Graham N, Lindesay J, Katona C et al, Reducing stigma and discrimination against older people with mental disorders: a technical consensus statement, *Int J Geriatr Psychiatry* (2003) **18**:670–8.

Haghighat R, A unitary theory of stigmatisation: pursuit of self-interest and routes to destigmatisation, *Br J Psychiatry* (2001) **178**:207–15.

Hilton J, von Hippel W, Stereotypes, *Annu Rev Psychol* (1996) **47**:237–71.

Holmes P, Corrigan P, Williams P et al, Changing attitudes about schizophrenia, *Schizophr Bull* (1999) **25**:447–56.

Keane M, Acceptance vs. rejection: nursing students' attitudes about mental illness, *Perspect Psychiatr Care* (1991) **27**:13–18.

Kolodziej ME, Johnson BT, Interpersonal contact and acceptance of persons with psychiatric disorders: a research synthesis, *J Consult Clin Psychol* (1996) **64**:387–96.

Link BG, Mirotznik J, Cullen FT, The effectiveness of stigma coping orientations: can negative consequences of mental illness labelling be avoided?, *J Health Soc Behav* (1991) **32**:302–20.

Morrison JK, Becker RE, Bourgeois CA, Decreasing adolescents' fear of mental illness by means of demythologising, *Psychol Rep* (1979) **44**:855–9.

Ostman M, Kjellin L, Stigma by association: psychological factors in relatives of people with mental illness, *Br J Psychiatry* (2002) **181**:494–8.

Penn D, Guynan K, Daily T et al, Dispelling the stigma of schizophrenia: what sort of information is best?, *Schizophr Bull* (1994) **20**:567–78.

Penn DL, Kohlmaier JR, Corrigan PW, Interpersonal factors contributing to the stigma of schizophrenia: social skills, perceived attractiveness, and symptoms, *Schizophr Res* (2000) **45**:37–45.

Stuart H, Arboleda-Florez J, Community attitudes toward people with schizophrenia, *Can J Psychiatry* (2001) **46**:245–52.

Thompson K, Stigma and public health policy for schizophrenia, *Psychiatr Clin North Am* (2003) **26**:273–94.

United Nations, *Principles for the Protection of Persons with Mental Illness and for the Improvement of Mental Health Care*, Resolution 46/119, adopted by the United Nations General Assembly, December (1991).

Wolff G, Pathare S, Craig T et al, Public education for community care: a new approach, *Br J Psychiatry* (1996) **168**:441–7.

World Health Organization/World Psychiatric Association, *Reducing Stigma and Discrimination against Older People with Mental Disorders: a Technical Consensus Statement* (World Health Organization/World Psychiatric Association: Geneva, 2002).

Wright ER, Gronfein WP, Owens TJ, Deinstitutionalization, social rejection, and the self-esteem of former mental patients, *J Health Soc Behav* (2000) **41**:68–90.

Part III

Other psychotic disorders in the elderly

chapter 11

Psychotic symptoms in delirium

Ravi Bhat

Introduction

There are no clear definitions for the term psychosis. In Fish's textbook of psychopathology a person suffering from psychosis has been described as 'an individual who lacks insight, has the whole of his personality distorted by illness and constructs a false environment out of his subjective experiences' (Hamilton, 1985, p.11). This rather broad conceptualization has resonance with lay meanings of madness but in practice does not allow for clear distinctions to be made between psychotic and nonpsychotic disorders. In ICD-10 (WHO, 1992, p.3) psychosis is defined as 'simply indicating the presence of hallucinations, delusions, or a limited number of several abnormalities of behavior, such as gross excitement and overactivity, marked psychomotor retardation, and catatonic behavior'. This definition captures what many understand by the term psychosis in daily practice. Psychosis in this chapter will be taken to mean presence of delusions or hallucinations unless otherwise specified.

Delirium has long been recognized to be a form of madness – a madness associated with fever or physical illness (Lipowski, 1990, pp. 4–5). The words that denote this syndrome reflect this understanding. The term delirium stems from the Latin word *delirare*, which literally means to go out of the furrow (*lira*, Latin for furrow) but whose vernacular meaning is to be deranged, crazy, out of one's wits (Lipowski, 1990, p.3). Another word used by the ancients was phrenitis, where the Greek words *phrén* or *phrenos* refer to both the diaphragm and the mind. The Greek word *phreneticos* means frenzied, frantic or mad.

Delirium as a cause of psychosis in the elderly

Delirium is common and often under-recognized in the elderly (Rockwood and Lindesay, 2002). While it is true that most of the studies have been hospital-based, studies in other settings also suggest a high prevalence. A recently published prevalence study of admission to post-acute facilities found a rate of 16%, with even more patients having sub-syndromal symptoms of delirium (Kiely et al, 2003). Prevalence of delirium was found to be 34% in home medical care and 58% in nursing homes in a large Swedish study (Bucht et al, 1999). In those diagnosed to have delirium only 24% had the diagnoses documented. Similar rates were found in an earlier Swedish study – 62% and 32% in nursing homes and old people's homes respectively (Dehlin and Franzen, 1985). A community study of nondemented oldest old found 10% of the people to have delirium (Rahkonen et al, 2001). Delirium has traditionally been thought to be a transient reversible condition; however, a review of outcome studies suggests that this is often not the case (Bhat and Rockwood, 2002). Psychotic symptoms are a part of the clinical presentation of delirium, occurring in approximately half of patients with delirium. Given the high rate of delirium in the elderly in various settings and its ability to persist for longer periods, it is reasonable to suppose that delirium might be a more common cause of psychotic symptoms in the elderly than is generally acknowledged (e.g. Mintzer and Targum, 2003).

This view is supported by a number of studies. In a prospective study Holroyd and Laurie (1999) evaluated 140 consecutive referrals of patients aged 60 and over to a geriatric psychiatry outpatient clinic; 27% of patients were found to have psychotic symptoms. Patients with psychosis were more likely to have delirium, dementia or organic psychosis (organic hallucinosis, organic delusional disorder) according to DSM-IIIR (American Psychiatric Association, 1987). The following four diagnoses explained nearly 80% of diagnoses in the psychotic group: dementia (36.4%), major depression (20.4%), delirium (12.2%), and other organic psychosis (10.2%). Typical psychiatric causes of psychosis such as schizophrenia, delusional disorders, etc. were relatively uncommon. Likewise, studies of patients being admitted to nursing homes and geriatric psychiatry wards have found that dementia, delirium, and organic psychosis were the commonest causes of psychosis in the elderly (Eastwood, 1983; Moriss et al, 1990).

Psychotic symptoms in delirium

There are not many studies of psychotic symptoms in delirium. Of the studies that have been published there are two kinds: those that have assessed patients cross-sectionally and those that have been done post delirium. Cross-sectional studies have often focused on rates of psychotic symptoms rather than the descriptive psychopathology. Even so, Meagher and Trzepacz (1998) in reviewing the psychopathology in delirium remark that very few papers report individual frequency of symptoms, with thought disorder and language dysfunction receiving extremely limited focus. Most of the post-delirium studies are phenomenological studies of delirium that provide some insights into the experience of delirium.

Meagher and Trzepacz (1998) found delusions to be as common as perceptual disturbances in the studies they reviewed. Delusions occurred in 18–68% of the patients; perceptual changes and/or hallucinations in 17–55%; and disorganized thinking or thought disorder in 95% of the patients. A Swedish study by Sandberg et al (1999) found that 315 of 717 patients were suffering from delirium. Psychotic symptoms occurred in 43.3% of the delirious patients; 28% of patients with hyperactive delirium suffered hallucinations or illusions and 31% experienced delusions compared with patients with hypoactive delirium, 15% of whom presented with hallucinations or illusions and 12.5% of whom had delusions. They also refer to paranoiac symptoms but these are not clearly defined in their paper. These occurred more commonly in patients with hyperactive delirium (47%) and in those delirious patients receiving home medical care than in patients in emergency hospital care, nursing homes, or old people's homes.

A retrospective study of delirium in 820 consecutive psychiatry consultations from medical and surgical wards found 227 patients with delirium (Webster and Holroyd, 2000); 42.7% of these patients had psychotic symptoms. Nearly 16% had both delusions and hallucinations; 32.6% had hallucinations, of whom 27% had visual hallucinations, 12.4% had auditory hallucinations, and 2.7% had tactile hallucinations; 26% had delusions, of which paranoid delusions were the commonest. This study found that only multiple etiologies were associated with psychotic symptoms in general, and visual hallucinations in particular. More than half the patients with delirium had a past history of a psychiatric illness but no single diagnosis was associated with psychotic symptoms in delirium.

Studies of delirium experience show that more than 50% of patients recall the delirium experience (Laitinen, 1996; Schoefield, 1997; Andersson et al, 2002; Breitbart et al, 2002a). In a quantitative study of 101 of 154 patients with cancer, Breitbart et al (2002a) found that in a logistical regression model, following short-term memory score and delirium severity, perceptual disturbances were associated with poor recall. Only 40% of patients with severe perceptual disturbance were able to recall versus 79% of those with either no or mild perceptual disturbance. Likewise presence of delusions too was negatively associated with recall (47% versus 71%). However, in those who did remember the delirium experience severity of perceptual disturbances and delusions positively correlated with delirium-related patient distress. Interestingly, other aspects of delirium such as severity, etc. were not positively correlated with distress. In a logistic regression model only delusions emerged as predictors of distress. It is likely that the severity of delirium correlates with poor recall rather than psychopathology itself.

Apart from delusions and hallucinations, manic symptoms may also be present in delirium or may follow delirium. Weintraub and Lippmann (2001) have reported two cases of delirious mania, a condition first described by Bell in 1849. Both the patients had past history of bipolar disorder and they first presented with signs of delirium that later evolved into manic symptoms. In 1909 Bonhoeffer also described a 66-year-old male who developed delirium following head injury evolving into a 'pronounced manic state' after the delirium subsided. These reports should be juxtaposed with the report that in some instances delirium might relieve psychosis (Malur et al, 2000). These authors reported six cases (patients aged 53–69) where an incidental delirium upon resolution successfully improved the mental state of the psychosis for which they had been admitted. The authors argue that following delirium the brain's self-regulatory mechanisms rectify pre-existing disorders.

In summary, psychotic symptoms appear to present in somewhat less than half of the patients suffering from delirium and appear to be the major cause of distress in those who could recall the delirium experience. Despite this, psychotic symptoms are not given prominence in clinical descriptions in classificatory systems such as DSM-IV (American Psychiatric Association, 1994). In fact delusions are not even mentioned as of one the features of delirium in DSM-IV.

Inter-relationship between symptoms, subtypes, and etiology

Studies of delirium symptoms indicate associations among cognitive function and delusions, hallucinations, psychomotor disturbances, sleep-wake changes, and mood lability (Meagher and Trzepacz, 1998). There were also associations between psychomotor disturbances and delusions, mood lability, and sleep changes and between hallucinations and mood lability. There was little correlation between hallucinations and delusions in one study. However, an interpretation of these studies is limited by the small sample sizes. One study examining the natural history of delirium found considerable heterogeneity (Rudberg et al, 1997). There is thus little research evidence about stability or persistence of symptoms in delirium, although clinical wisdom holds that symptoms are often transient.

Delirium has been classified into the hyperactive/hyperalert, hypoactive/hypoalert, and mixed subtypes (Lipowski, 1990). In their study Ross et al (1991) classified 58 patients into 'somnolent' and 'activated' subtypes on the basis of independent clinical interviews and analog scales. The activated patients had more hallucinations, delusions, and illusions on examination than somnolent patients and also had more hallucinatory and delusional behaviors in the two days prior to examination. Another study of 46 patients found that delusions, sleep-wake cycle disturbances, mood lability, and variability of symptoms distinguished between the hyperactive and hypoactive groups (Meagher et al, 2000). Psychotic symptoms appear to occur with a greater frequency in those suffering with hyperactive/hyperalert delirium.

The relationship between etiology and symptom profile is unclear because studies have usually examined the relationship between subtype and etiology. In the study quoted above by Meagher et al (2000), the authors found that delirium in closed head injuries and anticholinergic drug exposure was more likely to be hyperactive, and delirium due to metabolic causes and alcohol withdrawal was more likely to be hypoactive (Meagher and Trzepacz, 1998). The study of Ross et al (1991) also found that medication-related delirium was hyperactive and infectious and metabolic causes were hypoactive. However, O'Keeffe and Lavan (1999) did not find any etiological association with subtypes, although those with hypoactive delirium were more physically ill at admission. Any interpretation of association between symptoms, subtypes, and etiology is also made difficult by the fact that mixed subtype is the most common presentation of delirium.

Meaning of psychotic symptoms in delirium

There are three studies that have used phenomenological-hermeneutic methods to elucidate the delirium experience. These qualitative methodologies are based on Heideggerian philosophy and explore the meaning of experience (Crist and Tanner, 2003). These studies were carried out with the idea that understanding personal meaning can assist nurses in appropriately managing delirious patients. However, they also provide a window into understanding the development of psychotic symptoms in delirium and perhaps lead to development of models of delirium evolution and abnormal belief formation.

A small study of delirium experience in 19 elderly patients found that hallucinations (both visual and auditory) were common (Schoefield, 1997). They were often remembered as unpleasant, sinister and frightening with a few remembered as pleasant. Schoefield (1997) comments that one of the striking features was the intense feeling of reality of the delirium experience and yet having a sense of detachment – a quality that is reminiscent of the experience of dreams. A study by Laitinen (1996) also remarks on the insecurity of not knowing the here and now and loss of control, with feelings of reality and unreality at the same time.

A recent larger study by Andersson et al (2002) of 50 elderly patients with acute confusional state has confirmed and elaborated on some of these ideas. These authors found that most people felt trapped in incomprehensible experiences and the turmoil of past, present and here and there. In such states patients simultaneously encountered past, present and the realm of imagination as reality. However, while these experiences were apprehended as real and existing they were also seen as unreal and nonexistent. These descriptions are not new. Greiner, in his descriptions of delirium spoke of a blurring of the distinction between past and present (Lipowski, 1990). The patient might believe that dead persons he knew in the past were alive and speak to them, yet fail to recognize those familiar to him and present at his bedside (Lipowski, 1990).

Fleminger (2002), commenting on a psychiatrist's personal account of delirium, remarks that retrospective accounts, while as important as contemporaneous accounts, may be of questionable reliability. This is so because these could be retrospective constructions of remembered islets of psychotic experiences. The study of Andersson et al (2002) has to some extent overcome that problem by interviewing patients through their delirium rather than restricting their interpretations to just one post-delirium interview.

These accounts of delirium offer a view into the distorted and mixed perception of reality from which the rise of fragmented delusions is understandable – in the Jasperian sense of the term. It would also suggest that perhaps the abnormality of the delirium experience is an inability to integrate present, past and imaginary experiences and where (to paraphrase Fish) 'the individual lacks insight, has the whole of his personality distorted by illness and constructs a false environment out of his subjective experiences' (Hamilton, 1985, p.11).

Differential diagnoses

The differential diagnoses of delirium in the presence of psychotic symptoms would include many of the functional and organic psychoses in the elderly, including the dementias. Dementia is a risk factor for delirium and in 28–82% of cases delirium may be superimposed on dementia (Fick et al, 2002). Distinguishing between the two conditions can be difficult but abrupt changes in mental state or new-onset visual hallucinations in a person with known dementia may be indicative of a delirium in dementia.

Among the dementias the most important one is dementia with Lewy bodies (DLB). Delirium and DLB are psychopathologically very similar; both have a fluctuating impairment in consciousness with potentially multimodal hallucinations and presence of delusions (see Table 11.1). Visual hallucinations have generally been regarded as one of the characteristics of DLB; likewise new development of visual hallucinations in the elderly, especially the demented elderly, has been suggested to represent delirium. A comparison of visual hallucinations shows that there is greater similarity between DLB and delirium and that both these entities are different from hallucinations in other states such as Parkinson's disease, Charles-Bonnet syndrome, and late-onset schizophrenia (Barnes and David, 2001) (see Table 11.2).

Etiology, natural history, and treatment response may act as guides in distinguishing between these two disorders. Delirium is typically acute in onset with an identifiable cause or causes that may be associated with abnormal laboratory tests. However, laboratory tests may not be always be abnormal and as having had delirium once is itself a risk factor for future delirium one might get a history of multiple episodes of deliria confusing the picture. Sometimes follow-up may be the only way to differentiate the two conditions. Delirium does not appear to evolve into DLB on follow-up, even though available data on long-term follow-up of delirium suggests that dementia is

Table 11.1 Differential diagnoses of psychotic symptoms in delirium

Clinical features	Delirium	Dementia with Lewy bodies	Dementia	Late-onset schizophrenia
Consciousness	Impaired	Impaired	Usually not impaired but is in sundowning	Not impaired
Delusions	18–68%; often fragmented	47.6%	16–44%; delusions of theft, reference, strangers in the house	85%; persecution, reference, misidentification, control, primary
Auditory hallucinations	27%	14.3%	1–16%	50%
Visual hallucinations	12.4%	33%	4.4–32%	40%
Other hallucinations	–	–	–	30%; olfactory, touch or taste
Affective responses	43–63%	38% depressed	–	Preserved
Insight	Absent? Simultaneous or fluctuating awareness	Absent	Absent	Absent

Based on Ballard et al (1997); Meagher and Trzepacz (1998); Howard (1999); McKeith (2000); and Barnes and David (2001).

more likely to develop (reviewed in Bhat and Rockwood, 2002). Instead, a small study appears to suggest that the post-delirium dementia is more likely to be vascular dementia (Rahkonen et al, 2001). Haloperidol is often the treatment of choice in treating psychotic symptoms in delirium but causes significant extrapyramidal symptoms (EPS) in DLB and may be potentially fatal in that condition.

Table 11.2 Differential diagnoses of visual hallucinations in delirium

Psychopathological features of visual hallucinations	Delirium	Dementia with Lewy bodies	Charles-Bonnet syndrome/ Parkinson's disease
Background illumination	Usually dim	Unclear	Usually dim
State of consciousness	Often impaired	Often impaired	Alert
Eyes open or closed	Not known	Not known	Eyes open
Complex or elementary	Complex and elementary	Complex	Complex
Multimodal or not	? Multimodal	Often multimodal	Less often
Other hallucinations	Present – auditory	Present – auditory	Often absent
Moving or stationary	Often moving	Often moving	Moving
Transient or persistent	Often transient	Often persistent	Often transient
Form	? Fragmented	Complete	Complete
Meaningfulness	Often meaningful	Unclear	May be meaningful
Visions of dead?	Often	Unclear	Sometimes
Distress/perceived threat	Often distressing and/or threatening	Unclear	Usually nonthreatening
Insight	Usually absent	Usually absent	Usually present

Based on Lipowski (1990); McKeith (2000); Teunisse et al (1996); and Barnes and David (2001).

Mood disorders in late life constitute another group of disorders to be distinguished from delirium. Severe depression in late life can resemble both subtypes of delirium when it presents with psychomotor agitation or retardation. Other symptoms of such depression include poor sleep, impaired concentration, and psychotic symptoms. Collateral history of past episodes of depression and relatively gradual onset are important pointers to depression (Koponen et al, 2002). Mania with agitation, distractibility, and psychotic features can resemble delirium. Mania can also have atypical presentations as in delirious mania (Weintraub and Lippmann, 2001). Past history of bipolar disorder is important; however, in its absence late-onset mania is known to be more associated with organic factors.

Management

This section will concentrate on treatment of psychotic symptoms in delirium rather than management principles of delirium. The latter issues are dealt with in detail in specialist textbooks (see Marcantonio, 2002). The evidence base for pharmacologic treatment of delirium is not strong and is based on clinical experience, case reports, and review articles rather than randomized controlled trials (Cole et al, 1998). High potency antipsychotics such as haloperidol are considered the drugs of choice, as they do not have significant anticholinergic or sedative properties (Marcantonio, 2002). The dictum 'start low go slow' applies and haloperidol may be given from 0.5 to 3.0 mg/day in divided doses. When used in these doses it is preferable to use either twice a day or three times a day on a regular basis rather than *pro re nata*, as the latter runs the risk of unregulated use of higher doses leading to over-sedation. Haloperidol in doses greater than 3 mg/day may be associated with greater risk of EPS (Marcantonio, 2002). Apart from parkinsonian adverse effects, haloperidol may also cause akathisia. Akathisia causes significant distress and may be mistaken for worsening of a hyperactive delirium. In the latter event an increase in antipsychotic agent will just serve to worsen the akathisia rather than relieve delirium.

The advent of second-generation antipsychotics (SGAs) and their relatively lower potential to cause EPS has led to reports of their use in delirium. There are as yet no randomized controlled trials, with all reports either being case reports or open-label trials of risperidone, olanzapine quetiapine, and ziprasidone. Case reports of risperidone use have described it to be well tolerated in the elderly with delirium (Schwartz and Masand, 2002). A small prospective open trial of risperidone used in low doses (average 1.7 mg/day) in 10 patients with delirium found it to be effective in 80% of patients but 30% developed sedation and 10% developed mild drug-induced parkinsonism (Horikawa et al, 2003). Risperidone is available in tablets, liquid, and a dispersible formulation.

Absence of a short-acting injectable preparation is probably a limitation for use in emergencies. On average olanzapine appears to have a lower EPS risk than risperidone, although it has a greater anticholinergic potential and a greater potential to worsen diabetes. However, a large open trial of olanzapine in cancer patients with delirium found it to be effective and well tolerated (Breitbart et al, 2002b). Olanzapine is available in a wafer form and as a rapid-acting injectable preparation. Ziprasidone (Leso and Schwartz, 2002) and Quetiapine (mean dose around 90 mg/day for a mean of six days) (Kim et al, 2003) have both been described in case reports with no significant adverse effects.

While SGAs have a lower likelihood of EPS than first-generation antipsychotics (FGAs) they are not free of adverse effects. SGAs are also thought to be associated with an increased risk of obesity, diabetes, and dyslipidemia (American Diabetes Association et al, 2004). They are also known to exacerbate diabetes. Despite limitations in study design, the data consistently show an increased risk for diabetes in patients treated with clozapine or olanzapine compared with patients not receiving treatment with FGAs or with other SGAs (American Diabetes Association et al, 2004). Generalizability may be difficult when these drugs are used for relatively short periods as one would in treating delirium. However, the potential to worsen diabetes should be factored in when treating delirious elderly patients who have diabetes or who present with diabetic ketoacidosis.

Nonpharmacologic treatments in delirium often focus on increasing familiarity of people and surroundings and reorientation. The phenomenological studies (Laitinen, 1996; Schoefield, 1997; Andersson et al, 2002) offer some clues of how we could modify our behavior. Stability appears to be important, where the person feels secure by the mere presence of nursing staff. Staff should avoid using unnecessary jargon and talking among themselves in front of the patient any more than is absolutely necessary, especially when the patient's first language is not that of the staff.

Future directions

Delirium is one of the commonest causes of psychosis in the elderly; however, not much is known about the nature and course of psychotic symptoms in delirium. Prospective studies of descriptive psychopathology of delirium are needed along with comparative studies between delirium and DLB.

Frail elderly patients can be conceptualized as complex systems at the edge of failure, and when they fail, they will fail with their highest order functions first. For many patients, the highest order function will be consciousness, and thus their presentation will be delirium (Rockwood and Bhat, 2004). Impairment in consciousness is unlikely to be unidimensional, i.e. measurable only on a continuum of alertness to coma or manifest mainly as attentional impairment. More phenomenological studies are needed to replicate and clarify the delirium experience, for these can cast light on the nature of disturbance in consciousness in delirium and may also provide an understanding of abnormal belief formation in general.

Charlton and Kavanau (2002) have another view of the role of delirium in so-called functional psychiatric disorders. They suggest that although the current definition of delirium is parsimonious and prevents false positives in diagnosis it carries the implication that significant but mild delirium is probably routinely under-diagnosed. They hypothesize that serial EEGs would confirm that delirium is responsible for severe psychotic symptoms in many patients, particularly those with severe sleep loss or disruption. Greiner (quoted in Lipowski, 1990) considered that delirium (along with dreams) might offer deep insights into the innermost life of human beings. It is perhaps time that in daily practice we stopped 'thinking separately of organic and functional disorders' (Chiu and Ames, 1994, p.i) and in the process make delirium the focus of more systematic psychiatric research.

References

American Diabetes Association, American Psychiatric Association, American Association of Clinical Endocrinologists, North American Association for the Study of Obesity, Consensus Development Conference on Antipsychotic Drugs and Obesity and Diabetes, *Diabetes Care* (2004) **27**:596–601.

American Psychiatric Association, *Diagnostic and Statistical Manual of Mental Disorders*, 3rd edn (revised) (DSM III R), (American Psychiatric Association: Washington, DC, 1987).

American Psychiatric Association, *Diagnostic and Statistical Manual of Mental Disorders*, 4th edn (DSM-IV) (American Psychiatric Association: Washington, DC, 1994).

Andersson EM, Hallberg IR, Norberg A, Edberg AK, The meaning of acute confusional state from the perspective of elderly patients, *Int J Geriatr Psychiatry* (2002) 17:652–63.

Ballard C, McKeith I, Harrison R et al, A detailed phenomenological comparison of complex visual hallucinations in dementia with Lewy bodies and Alzheimer's disease, *Int Psychogeriatrics* (1997) 9:381–8.

Barnes J, David AS, Visual hallucinations in Parkinson's disease: a review and phenomenological survey, *J Neurol Neurosurg Psychiatry* (2001) 70:727–33.

Bhat RS, Rockwood K, The prognosis of delirium, *Psychogeriatrics* (2002) 2:165–79.

Bonhoeffer K, Exogenous psychoses, *Zentralbleitt für Nervenheilkunde* (1909) 32:499–505. Translated by Marshall H, in: Hirsch SR, Shepherd M, eds, *Themes and Variations in European Psychiatry* (John Wright and Sons.: Bristol, 1974) 47–52.

Breitbart W, Gibson C, Tremblay A, The delirium experience: delirium recall and delirium-related distress in hospitalized patients with cancer, their spouses/caregivers, and their nurses, *Psychosomatics* (2002a) **43**:183–94.

Breitbart W, Tremblay A, Gibson C, An open trial of olanzapine for the treatment of delirium in hospitalized cancer patients, *Psychosomatics* (2002b) **43**:175–82.

Bucht G, Gustafson Y, Sandberg O, Epidemiology of delirium, *Dement Geriatr Cogn Disord* (1999) **10**:315–18.

Charlton BG, Kavanau JL, Delirium and psychotic symptoms – an integrative model, *Med Hypotheses* (2002) **58**:24–7.

Chiu E, Ames D, *Functional Psychiatric Disorders of the Elderly* (Cambridge University Press: Cambridge, 1994).

Cole MG, Primeau FJ, Élie ML, Delirium: prevention, treatment and outcome studies, *J Geriatr Psychiatry Neurol* (1998) **11**:126–37.

Crist JD, Tanner CA, Interpretation/analysis methods in hermeneutic interpretive phenomenology, *Nurs Res* (2003) **52**:202–5.

Dehlin O, Franzen M, Prevalence of dementia syndromes in persons living in homes for the elderly and in nursing homes in southern Sweden, *Scand J Prim Health Care* (1985) **3**:215–22.

Eastwood MR, Hallucinations in patients admitted to a geriatric psychiatry service: review of 42 cases, *J Am Geriatr Soc* (1983) **12**:251–61.

Fick DM, Agostini JV, Inouye SK, Delirium superimposed on dementia: a systematic review, *J Am Geriatr Soc* (2002) **50**:1723–32.

Fleminger S, Remembering delirium, *Br J Psychiatry* (2002) **180**:4–5.

Hamilton M, *Fish's Clinical Psychopathology: Signs and Symptoms in Psychiatry*, 2nd edn, (Wright: Bristol, 1985) 11–12.

Holroyd S, Laurie S, Correlates of psychotic symptoms among elderly outpatients, *Int J Geriatr Psychiatry* (1999) **14**:379–84.

Horikawa N, Yamazaki T, Miyamoto K et al, Treatment for delirium with risperidone: results of a prospective open trial with 10 patients, *Gen Hosp Psychiatry* (2003) **25**:289–92.

Howard R, Schizophrenia-like psychosis with onset in late life. In: Howard R, Rabins PV, Castle DJ, eds, *Late Onset Schizophrenia* (Wrightson Biomedical Publishing: Petersfield, 1999) 127–46.

Kiely DK, Bergmann MA, Murphy KM et al, Delirium among newly admitted postacute facility patients: prevalence, symptoms, and severity, *J Gerontol A Biol Sci Med Sci* (2003) **58**:M441–M445.

Kim KY, Bader GM, Kotlyar V, Gropper D, Treatment of delirium in older adults with quetiapine, *J Geriatr Psychiatry Neurol* (2003) **16**:29–31.

Koponen H, Rockwood K, Powell C, Clinical assessment and diagnosis. In: Lindesay J, Rockwood K, Macdonald A, eds, *Delirium in Old Age* (Oxford University Press: Oxford, 2002) 91–100.

Laitinen H, Patients' experience of confusion in the intensive care unit following cardiac surgery, *Intensive Crit Care Nurs* (1996) **12**:79–83.

Leso L, Schwartz TL, Ziprasidone treatment of delirium, *Psychosomatics* (2002) **43**:61–2.

Lipowski ZJ, *Delirium: Acute Confusional States* (Oxford University Press: New York, 1990).

Malur C, Fink M, Fracis A, Can delirium relieve psychosis?, *Compr Psychiatry* (2000) **41**:450–3.

Marcantonio E, The management of delirium. In: Lindesay J, Rockwood K, Macdonald A, eds, *Delirium in Old Age* (Oxford University Press: Oxford, 2002) 123–51.

McKeith I, Dementia with Lewy Bodies: a clinical overview. In: O'Brien J, Ames D, Burns A, eds, *Dementia* 2nd edn (Arnold: London, 2000) 685–97.

Meagher DJ, O'Hanlon D, O'Mahony E et al, Relationship between symptoms and motoric subtype of delirium, *J Neuropsychiatry Clin Neurosci* (2000) **12**:51–6.

Meagher DJ, Trzepacz PT, Delirium phenomenology illuminates pathophysiology, management, and course, *J Geriatr Psychiatry Neurol* (1998) **11**:150–6.

Mintzer J, Targum SD, Psychosis in elderly patients: classification and pharmacotherapy, *J Geriatr Psychiatry Neurol* (2003) **16**:199–206.

Moriss RK, Rovner BW, Folstein MF, German PS, Delusions in newly admitted residents of nursing homes, *Am J Psychiatry* (1990) **147**:299–302.

O'Keeffe ST, Lavan JN, Clinical significance of delirium subtypes in older people, *Age Ageing* (1999) **28**:115–19.

Rahkonen T, Eloniemi-Sulkava U, Halonen P et al, Delirium in the non-demented oldest old in the general population: risk factors and prognosis, *Int J Geriatr Psychiatry* (2001) **16**:415–21.

Rockwood K, Bhat RS, Should we think before we treat delirium?, *Int Med J* (2004) **34**: 76–8.

Rockwood K, Lindesay J, The concept of delirium: historical antecedents and present meanings. In: Lindesay J, Rockwood K, Macdonald A, eds, *Delirium in Old Age* (Oxford University Press: Oxford, 2002) 1–8.

Ross CA, Peyser CE, Shapiro I et al, Delirium: phenomenologic and etiologic subtypes, *Int Psychogeriatrics* (1991) **3**:135–47.

Rudberg MA, Pompei P, Foreman MD et al, The natural history of delirium in older hospitalized patients: a syndrome of heterogeneity, *Age Ageing* (1997) **26**:169–74.

Sandberg O, Gustafson Y, Braennstroem B, Bucht G, Clinical profile of delirium in older patients, *J Am Geriatr Soc* (1999) **47**:1300–6.

Schoefield I, A small exploratory study of the reaction of older people to an episode of delirium, *J Adv Nurs* (1997) **25**:942–52.

Schwartz TL, Masand PS, The role of atypical antipsychotics in the treatment of delirium, *Psychosomatics* (2002) **43**:171–4.

Teunisse RJ, Cruysberg JR, Hoefnagels WH et al, Visual hallucinations in psychologically normal people: Charles Bonnet's syndrome, *Lancet* (1996) **347**:794–7.

Webster R, Holroyd S, Prevalence of psychotic symptoms in delirium, *Psychosomatics* (2000) **41**:519–22.

Weintraub D, Lippmann S, Delirious mania in the elderly, *Int J Geriatr Psychiatry* (2001) **16**:374–7.

World Health Organization, *The ICD-10 Classification of Mental and Behavioural Disorders: Clinical Descriptions and Diagnostic Guidelines* (World Health Organization: Geneva, 1992).

chapter 12

Psychosis in affective disorders – depression

David Ames

What is psychotic depression?

Definitions of psychosis as they apply to older people have been addressed in Chapter 2. Psychosis is a difficult word to define (Bowman and Rose, 1951) and its usage in relation to late-life depression has varied depending upon the contexts and times in which it has been employed. Older classification systems tended to class all severe, endogenous, biological or melancholic type depressions as 'depressive psychosis' (Meyers, 1995), but more recent international nomenclatures have tended to reserve the term for those who have depression with co-morbid delusions, hallucinations or depressive stupor (Meyers, 1995).

The American Psychiatric Association's DSM-IV (1994) defines a major depressive episode (MDE) as being present when the patient has experienced for two weeks or more, five or more depressive symptoms, which comprise: depressed mood, markedly diminished interest or pleasure in activities, significant weight loss or gain or change in appetite, insomnia/hypersomnia, psychomotor retardation or agitation, fatigue or loss of energy, feelings of worthlessness or excessive or inappropriate guilt, diminished ability to think or concentrate or indecisiveness, and recurrent thoughts of death, suicide or a suicidal attempt or plan. The symptoms must not meet criteria for a mixed episode, must cause clinically significant distress or impairment, cannot be due to the direct effects of substance abuse or a general medical condition and must not be better accounted for by bereavement. Either depressed mood or loss of interest or pleasure must be among the expressed symptoms to permit the diagnosis to be made. Various levels of severity are defined in the manual including an episode which is 'severe with psychotic features'. Such an episode is characterized as exhibiting 'delusions or hallucinations'. If possible, specify whether the psychotic features are mood-congruent or mood-incongruent:

- **Mood-congruent psychotic features:** Delusions or hallucinations whose content is entirely consistent with the typical depressive themes of personal inadequacy, guilt, disease, death, nihilism, or deserved punishment.
- **Mood-incongruent psychotic features:** Delusions or hallucinations whose content does not involve typical depressive themes of personal inadequacy, guilt, disease, death, nihilism, or deserved punishment. Included are such symptoms as persecutory delusions (not directly related to depressive themes), thought insertion, thought broadcasting, and delusions of control.'

An episode with psychotic features is presumed to be severe – no specifiers are listed for a MDE with psychotic features which is not of severe degree.

The diagnostic criteria for research of the World Health Organization's ICD-10 system (WHO, 1992) permit the diagnosis of a severe depressive episode with psychotic features when at least eight of the following 10 symptoms are present: depressed mood abnormal for the individual, loss of interest or pleasure in normally pleasurable activities, decreased energy or fatiguability, loss of confidence/self-esteem, unreasonable self-reproach/guilt, recurrent thoughts of death or suicide or suicidal behavior, diminished ability to think or concentrate, psychomotor agitation/retardation, sleep disturbance, change in appetite with weight change. Each of the first three symptoms must be expressed, the episode must not exhibit manic symptoms, should not be attributable to substance use or organic mental disorder and must have lasted for at least two weeks. In addition there must be either:

'1. Delusions or hallucinations . . . other than those . . . typically schizophrenic. The commonest examples are those with depressive, guilty, hypochondriacal, nihilistic or persecutory content.
2. Depressive stupor.'

Provision is made for specification of the psychotic symptoms as congruent (e.g. delusions of guilt, worthlessness, bodily disease or impending disaster, derisive or condemnatory auditory hallucinations) or incongruent (e.g. persecutory or self-referential delusions or hallucinations without an affective content) with the mood. Depressive stupor is not defined. Again no provision is made for the classification as psychotic of depressive episodes which are mild or moderate in severity.

A somewhat more traditional approach to the classification of depressive psychosis is apparent in the GMS-AGECAT computerized diagnostic system developed by Copeland et al (1986) and widely used in epidemiological research with the elderly. In this system an individual with depressive symptoms will be classed as a case of depressive psychosis if typical melancholic features such as depressed mood that is worse in the morning, inability to weep, morning slowness, early morning wakening, retardation, muddled thinking, and appetite and weight loss are present. However, if mood-congruent hallucinations or delusions are present, the subject will be diagnosed with depressive psychosis at the highest possible level of confidence (level 5), as opposed to levels 3 or 4, which are reserved for those with melancholic features lacking frank psychotic symptoms (Copeland et al, 1987).

In clinical samples of depressed patients with psychotic features, delusions are more common than hallucinations, which are not usually present except in combination with delusions (Meyers, 1995). However, in some community samples hallucinations are reported without delusions in a relatively large percentage of subjects experiencing a MDE and in an even larger proportion of individuals whose depressive symptoms do not meet MDE criteria (Ohayon and Schatzberg, 2002).

Debates about how best to classify depression have continued for over half a century (Kendall, 1976; Parker et al, 2003) and show no sign of abating. Some authorities suggest that depression with psychotic features should be considered as a separate disorder from other forms of depression (Meyers, 1995; Rothschild, 2003), while others who have reviewed the literature conclude that evidence for accepting psychotic depression in old age as a distinct entity is limited at best (Baldwin, 1992). Parker (2000) has argued – on the basis of meticulous research – that melancholia is a core depressive disorder surrounded by a penumbra of nonmelancholic conditions with depressive features and, through the analysis with colleagues of depressive symptoms seen in 123 elderly depressed patients referred for psychiatric treatment (Parker et al, 2003), has adduced evidence which favors a tripartite model for late-life depression which distinguishes psychotic, melancholic, and nonmelancholic subtypes. Nevertheless, it is safe to say that the tension between 'lumpers' and 'splitters' has not yet been resolved to the point where consensus is likely to break out in the immediate future!

What causes psychotic depression in late life?

Baldwin (2002) has compiled a thorough review of the putative etiologies of late-life depression and these will not be rehearsed in detail here. Only research which bears directly upon the question of the etiology of depression with psychotic features will be addressed. Most of this research has compared patients of all ages who have psychotic depression with nonpsychotic depressed subjects. Elderly patients have not been the specific focus of most studies, although most series include at least some elderly people. Many studies appearing to differentiate etiological risk factors for psychotic from nonpsychotic depression have not been widely replicated.

In some but not all studies which compare individuals with psychotic depression with depressed subjects lacking psychotic features, there is a higher rate of depression (Leckman et al, 1984; Nelson et al, 1984) and even of psychotic depression (Leckman et al, 1984) among the first-degree relatives of the psychotic subjects.

Individuals presenting with major depression at a relatively young age are more likely to exhibit mania later (i.e. to 'convert' from unipolar to bipolar affective disorder) if they have psychotic symptoms at baseline (Strober and Carlson, 1982; Akiksal et al, 1983).

There is evidence of hypothalamic-pituitary-adrenal axis dysfunction in people who have psychotic depression. A meta-analysis of 12 studies including more than 1000 patients found that psychosis rather than melancholic symptoms was associated with increased rates of nonsuppression of cortisol production by dexamethasone (Nelson and Davis, 1997). Activation of the dopaminergic system also may characterize individuals with psychotic depression (Schatzberg and Rothschild, 1992; Rothschild, 2003).

Some studies have reported brain imaging abnormalities in individuals with psychotic depression. Rothschild and colleagues (1989) found cognitive impairment that was associated with increased ventricle–brain ratio on CT (computed tomography) scan among depressed patients expressing psychotic symptoms. Decreased prefrontal cortex volumes were found when elderly patients experiencing a psychotic MDE were subjected to brain magnetic resonance imaging (MRI) scans and compared with patients experiencing a nonpsychotic MDE (Kim et al, 1999). On the other hand, despite increasing interest in the topic of vascular depression (Chiu et al, 2002), Krishnan et al (1997) actually found that depressed patients with hyperintensities seen on brain MRI were less likely to exhibit psychotic symptoms than depressed subjects lacking such lesions, while Sackeim (2001) concluded that there was no difference in the severity of MRI brain hyperintensities between patients with psychotic and nonpsychotic depression referred for electroconvulsive therapy (ECT).

At this stage, support from etiological studies for the concept of late-life psychotic depression as a separate entity from nonpsychotic depression must be considered weak at best. Existing data may be explained just as well by viewing depression as a single entity of varying degrees of severity in which psychotic symptoms are manifested only in the severe forms of the disorder.

Who has psychotic depression?

A limited number of epidemiologic studies have reported rates of depression with psychotic features among older adults living in the community. Copeland and colleagues (1987) found that 3% of 1070 elderly Liverpudlians fulfilled the diagnostic requirements of the GMS-AGECAT system for depressive psychosis, a broad category equivalent to melancholic or endogenous depression. However, only one elderly woman attained the highest level (5) of confidence for the depressive psychosis diagnosis, which is reached only if mood-congruent delusions or hallucinations are present. Many other studies have used GMS-AGECAT to report the prevalence of depression in community samples but most do not specify how many (if any) subjects were diagnosed with depressive psychosis at confidence level 5 (e.g. Saunders et al, 1993). In one report from nine European centres, GMS-AGECAT depressive psychosis prevalence ranged from 1.9% in Amsterdam to 10.6% in Munich and as a proportion of all case level depressions from just under 7% in Dublin to 45% in Munich (Copeland et al, 1999).

An epidemiologic study of depression among 1529 Finns aged above 60 found 42 to have a DSM-III MDE (American Psychiatric Association, 1980) and of these, three had hallucinatory depression and 12 had delusional symptoms, giving a point prevalence for males of 2/1000 for hallucinatory and 6/1000 for delusional depression, while for women the rates were 3/1000 and 12/1000, respectively (Kivelä and Pahkala, 1988, 1989).

There have been studies of psychotic depression in mixed age population samples too. In the United States Epidemiologic Catchment Area (ECA) study the lifetime rate for major depression was reported to be 4.4% among more than 18,000 adults from five cities, and 14.7% of these were thought to be psychotic cases, yielding a lifetime prevalence of psychotic depression of 0.6% (Johnson et al, 1991). Most (83%) of the individuals with a history of psychotic depression were female and their average age was 42. There was no significant age difference between psychotic and nonpsychotic depression subjects, but the former were more likely to report multiple episodes of depression (74% vs 62%), were twice as likely (27% vs 13%) to report a history of attempted suicide, and also had a higher lifetime psychiatric hospitalization rate (23% vs 15%), although the rate still seems astonishingly low, casting considerable doubt on whether what was being diagnosed here would be recognized as depression with psychotic symptoms by clinicians used to dealing with clinical populations. The methodology and findings of the ECA study have been robustly criticized (Burvill, 1987; Snowdon, 1990).

A European study of 18,980 subjects from five countries aged from 15 to 100 and interviewed by telephone reported a current prevalence of MDE with psychotic features of 0.4% (95% CI 0.35–0.54%) (Ohayon and Schatzberg, 2002). Of the 2.4% of the total sample who had a current MDE, 18.5% had psychotic symptoms. Hallucinations (97% auditory) were somewhat less common (6.8% of major depression subjects) than delusions (10.6% of major depression subjects) and only 1.2% of those with major depression had both delusions and hallucinations. Age had no significant effect upon risk for psychotic depression (0.3% of those aged above 65, 95% CI 0.1–0.5%) but rates of nonpsychotic depression were significantly lower among those aged 65 and over (1.3%, 95% CI 0.9–1.7%). Once again rates of treatment were extremely low for what seems to be in clinical practice a severe and disabling illness, but they were higher for those with psychotic major depression of whom 28% had consulted a health professional for treatment of depression in the past compared with 18% of those with nonpsychotic major depression. Women were more likely to have both psychotic and nonpsychotic depression than men (0.6% vs 0.3% female:male ratio for psychotic, 2.3% vs 1.6% for nonpsychotic).

Studies of depressed elderly subjects presenting for (usually inpatient) treatment are biased by differential rates of referral and admission based on symptom severity, cost of treatment and access to inpatient beds. Rates of psychotic depression in such clinical samples vary from a low of 24% (Murphy, 1983), through 40% of those with a MDE (Parker et al, 2003) to 45% (Meyers and Greenberg, 1986) and even 53% (Post, 1972).

A significant number of community-dwelling elderly people with depression can be expected to exhibit psychotic symptoms and these symptoms will be encountered frequently among the depressed elderly presenting for treatment.

How should we treat psychotic depression in the elderly?

There is evidence to indicate that psychotic depression responds to electro-convulsive therapy (ECT). In a combined analysis of the Leicester and Northwick Park randomized controlled ECT trials depressed patients with retardation and delusions did better with real than with simulated ECT, while depressed patients who were neither retarded nor deluded did no better with real ECT (Buchan et al, 1992). The presence of delusions was associated with increased response to ECT in a cohort of elderly patients (Mulsant et al, 1991) and in a prognostic study of late-life depression where ECT was used sparingly the presence of delusions was predictive of poor outcome (Murphy, 1983), whereas this was not the case in another study reporting higher usage of ECT (Baldwin and Jolley, 1986). However, in a retrospective analysis of 135 elderly depressed patients treated at three hospitals, Gormley et al (1999) found no difference in response between depressed patients with or without psychotic features, although ECT was effective in treating both groups of patients. Psychotic depression responds better to treatment with ECT than to drug treatment (Pande et al, 1990; Parker et al, 1992; Flint and Rifat, 1998), although one review of 17 studies of delusional depression (Kroessler, 1985) found only a slight advantage for ECT over the combination of an anti-depressant and an antipsychotic (82% vs 75% response in 597 patients). It may be that selection biases including earlier treatment with ECT for psychotic depressed patients and later selection for ECT after pharmacotherapy has failed, may exaggerate the efficacy of ECT for late-life psychotic depression, while the comparison of ECT with a variety of medication regimes makes conclusions about its advantage over specific regimes hard to reach. Nevertheless, over 66 years ECT has set a standard for the acute treatment of psychotic depression that pharmacotherapy has yet to match, and guidelines for the treatment of depression in older people endorse its use as first-line treatment in elderly patients with psychotic depression (Baldwin et al, 2002).

Early depression treatment studies with tricyclic antidepressants revealed inferior outcomes for psychotic depressed patients, many of whom went on later to improve with ECT (Rothschild, 2003). The trials which established the selective serotonin reuptake inhibitors (SSRIs) as effective treatments for depression specifically excluded delusional subjects from treatment. A series of studies from Italy (Gatti et al, 1996; Zanardi et al, 1996, 2000) have reported good outcomes in psychotic depression patients treated with SSRI or selective serotonin and noradrenaline reuptake inhibitor (SNRI) mono-therapy, but the studies lacked a placebo control arm, used a rating scale of questionable validity, and have not been replicated by other researchers (Rothschild and Phillips, 1999). Open-label studies of amoxapine in the treatment of psychotic depression also showed encouraging recovery rates of 60–80% (Anton and Sexauer, 1983).

The best evidence for the efficacy of pharmacotherapy in late-life psychotic depression comes from studies which have assessed use of a combination of antidepressant and antipsychotic drug treatment (Mulsant et al, 2001; Rothschild, 2003). However, current American Psychiatric Association (2000) guidelines which endorse the use of an antipsychotic in combination with an antidepressant for the initial treatment of a psychotic MDE are based on one study which found that of 58 deluded patients with a MDE, 19% recovered on perphenazine alone, 41% on monotherapy with amitriptyline, and 78% got well using a combination of both drugs (Spiker et al, 1985). A later trial by Anton and Burch (1990) reported impressive recovery rates of 71% and 81% for psychotic MDE patients treated with amoxapine alone or a combination of amitriptyline and perphenazine, respectively. However, Mulsant and colleagues (2001) did not find that the addition of perphenazine to nortriptyline improved outcome in elderly psychotic MDE patients at all. Atypical antipsychotic therapy has been examined in two important studies. Muller-Siecheneder et al (1998) found the combination of haloperidol and amitriptyline to be superior to risperidone alone in producing improvement over six weeks of therapy in patients with psychotic depression, but risperidone use was associated with worthwhile reductions in symptom severity. Dubé et al (2002) randomized 249 psychotic MDE patients to treatment with olanzapine alone, fluoxetine plus olanzapine, or placebo. Over half of those on combined treatment improved, compared with just over and just under one-third of those on olanzapine monotherapy and placebo, respectively.

Important questions remain to be answered with regard to the use of pharmacotherapy as first-line treatment for psychotic depression, and some of these are being addressed by a high quality North American study currently in progress, which aims to randomize over 300 patients with a psychotic MDE to a variety of drug treatment parameters (Meyers et al, 2004).

It can be argued that the toughest challenge in the management of late-life depression in general and of psychotic late-life depression in particular, lies not in achieving recovery from an acute episode of illness, but in preventing recovered patients from relapsing (Ames and Allen, 1991). If the evidence base for the pharmacologic treatment of acute episodes of late-life psychotic depression may fairly be described as thin, then the body of knowledge in regard to relapse prevention is positively emaciated (Meyers et al, 2001). Inferences from follow-up studies of old patients with major depression suggest that prophylactic pharmacotherapy should be continued for between six months and the remainder of the lifespan, but clear guidance as to doses and the relative usefulness of individual antidepressants, antipsychotics, lithium, and even maintenance ECT is lacking (Baldwin et al, 2002; Meyers, 1995). Most old age psychiatrists would be reluctant to cease pharmacotherapy within less than two years of recovery from a psychotic MDE and many would use lithium prophylaxis in individuals who experience repeated relapses despite prophylactic antidepressant treatment. Prophylaxis against relapse using a variety of agents including lithium will be addressed in the National Institutes of Mental Health severe depression trial (Meyers et al, 2004).

What happens to old people with psychotic depression?

Old people treated for depression tend to relapse and have higher death rates than those who have never been depressed (Ames and Allen, 1991). Excellent reviews of the prognosis of depression in old age exist (Cole and Bellavance, 1997) and their contents will not be reiterated in detail here. Instead this section will focus upon the limited evidence which pertains to the long-term outcome of elderly patients who experience depression with psychotic features.

Murphy's (1983) finding that only 10% of elderly patients with delusional depression had a good one-year outcome has been alluded to above, as has the finding of Baldwin and Jolley (1986) that with higher rates of ECT, delusions did not predict a bad one-year outcome for late-life depression. However, Baldwin (1988) did find that deluded elderly depressed patients were more than twice as likely to require readmission over 3.5–5 years than their counterparts who were not deluded at baseline.

In a retrospective analysis of 25 years of experience with patients committing suicide who had previously undergone hospital treatment for depression, those who had delusions during the index depressive episode had five times the risk of completed suicide than did subjects who were not psychotic when first treated (Roose et al, 1983).

In a more recent long-term follow-up study (Vythilingam et al, 2003) a group of 61 psychotic depression patients (mean age = 63) were compared with 59 depression patients who had not been psychotic. The risk of mortality for the psychotic group was doubled (41% vs 20%) over 15 years of follow-up, even after allowing for age and medical status as covariates (hazards ratio 2.31).

Conclusions

Whether or not late-life psychotic depression represents a distinct clinical entity or merely the severe extreme of a spectrum of late-life depressive disorders, clinicians who treat elderly depressed patients will encounter many (between one-quarter and one-half of all inpatient referrals) who have psychotic features, most usually delusions. There may be a significant number of deluded depressed elderly people in the community who are not in contact with psychiatric services, although it is likely that the phenomenology of their disorders may be different from that of patients presenting to clinicians. Elderly patients with psychotic depression who present for treatment have a high risk of suicide and a low rate of spontaneous recovery and so their disorder should be treated aggressively. The best evidence for treatment efficacy in this condition lies with ECT. Prophylactic antidepressant therapy is recommended after recovery, but the ideal duration of such treatment is controversial, as is the question of whether it should be accompanied by an antipsychotic drug. There is considerable need for further research, particularly into the efficacy of various combinations of drug treatments for the acute illness and the ideal pharmacotherapy for long-term prophylaxis (Martinez et al, 1996).

References

Akiksal HS, Walker P, Puzantian VR et al, Bipolar outcome in the course of depressive illness: phenomenological, familial, and pharmacologic predictors, *J Affect Disord* (1983) 5:115–28.

American Psychiatric Association, *Diagnostic and Statistical Manual of Mental Disorders*, 3rd edn (DSM-III) (American Psychiatric Association: Washington, DC, 1980).

American Psychiatric Association, *Diagnostic and Statistical Manual of Mental Disorders*, 4th edn (DSM-IV) (American Psychiatric Association: Washington, DC, 1994).

American Psychiatric Association, Practice Guidelines for the treatment of major depressive disorder (revision), *Am J Psychiatry* (2000) 157 (Suppl 4).

Ames D, Allen N, The prognosis of depression in old age: good, bad or indifferent, *Int J Geriatr Psychiatry* (1991) 6:477–81.

Anton RF, Burch EA, Amoxapine versus amitriptyline combined with perphenazine in the treatment of psychotic depression, *Am J Psychiatry* (1990) **147**:1203–8.

Anton RF, Sexauer JD, Efficacy of amoxapine in psychotic depression, *Am J Psychiatry* (1983) **140**:1344–7.

Baldwin RC, Delusional and non-delusional depression in late life: evidence for distinct subtypes, *Br J Psychiatry* (1988) **152**:39–44.

Baldwin RC, The nature, prevalence and frequency of depressive delusions. In: Katona C, Levy R, eds, *Delusions and Hallucinations in Old Age* (Gaskell: London, 1992).

Baldwin RC, Depressive disorders. In: Jacoby R, Oppenheimer C, eds, *Psychiatry in the Elderly*, 3rd edn (Oxford University Press: Oxford, 2002) 627–76.

Baldwin RC, Jolley D, The prognosis of depression in old age, *Br J Psychiatry* (1986) **149**:574–83.

Baldwin RC, Chiu E, Katona C, Graham N, *Guidelines on Depression in Older People* (Martin Dunitz: London, 2002).

Bowman K, Rose M, A criticism of the terms 'psychosis', 'psychoneurosis' and 'neurosis', *Am J Psychiatry* (1951) **108**:161–6.

Buchan H, Johnstone E, McPherson K et al, Who benefits from electroconvulsive therapy? Combined results of the Leicester and Northwick Park Trials, *Br J Psychiatry* (1992) **160**:355–9.

Burvill PW, An appraisal of the NIMH epidemiologic catchment area program, *Aust N Z J Psychiatry* (1987) **21**:175–84.

Chiu E, Ames D, Katona C, *Vascular Disease and Affective Disorders* (Martin Dunitz: London, 2002).

Cole M, Bellavance F, The prognosis of depression in old age, *Am J Geriatr Psychiatry* (1997) **5**:4–14.

Copeland JRM, Dewey ME, Griffiths-Jones HM, Psychiatric case nomenclature and a computerised diagnostic system for elderly subjects: GMS and AGECAT, *Psychol Med* (1986) **16**:219–23.

Copeland JRM, Beekman ATF, Dewey ME et al, Depression in Europe: geographical distribution among older people, *Br J Psychiatry* (1999) **174**:312–21.

Copeland JRM, Dewey ME, Wood N et al, Range of mental illness among the elderly in the community: prevalence in Liverpool using the GMS-AGECAT package, *Br J Psychiatry* (1987) **150**:815–23.

Dubé S, Andersen SW, Sanger TM et al, Olanzapine-fluoxetine combination for psychotic major depression. Poster presented at the *157th Annual Meeting of the American Psychiatric Association*, Philadelphia, USA, May 18–23 (2002).

Flint A, Rifat SL, The treatment of psychotic depression in later life: a comparison of pharmacotherapy and ECT, *Int J Geriatr Psychiatry* (1998) **13**:23–8.

Gatti F, Elini L, Gasperini M et al, Fluvoxamine alone in the treatment of delusional depression, *Am J Psychiatry* (1996) **153**:414–16.

Gormley N, Cullen C, Watters L et al, Does psychosis predict response to ECT in depressed elderly patients?, *Ir J Psych Med* (1999) **16**:13–15.

Johnson J, Horwath E, Weissman MM, The validity of major depression with psychotic features based on a community sample, *Arch Gen Psychiatry* (1991) **48**:1075–81.

Kendall R, The classification of depressions: a review of contemporary confusion, *Br J Psychiatry* (1976) **129**:15–28.

Kim DK, Kim BL, Sohn SE et al, Candidate neuroanatomic substrates of psychosis in old-aged depression, *Prog Neuropsychopharmacol Biol Psychiatry* (1999) **23**:793–807.

Kivelä S-L, Pahkala K, Hallucinatory depression in the elderly: a community study, *Z Altenforsch* (1988) **43**:331–9.

Kivelä S-L, Pahkala K, Delusional depression in the elderly, a community study, *Z Gerontol* (1989) **22**:236–41.

Krishnan KR, Hays JC, Blazer DG, MRI defined vascular depression, *Am J Psychiatry* (1997) **154**:497–501.

Kroessler D, Relative efficacy rates for therapies of delusional depression, *Convulsive Ther* (1985) **1**:173–82.

Leckman JF, Weisman MM, Prusoff BA et al, Subtypes of depression: family study perspective, *Arch Gen Psychiatry* (1984) **41**:833–8.

Martinez RA, Mulsant BH, Meyers BS, Lebowitz BD, Delusional and psychotic depression in late life: clinical research needs, *Am J Geriatr Psychiatry* (1996) **4**:77–84.

Meyers BS, Late-life delusional depression: acute and long-term treatment, *Int Psychogeriatrics* (1995) **7**(Suppl):113–24.

Meyers BS, Greenberg R, Late-life delusional depression, *J Affect Disord* (1986) **11**:133–7.

Meyers BS, Klimstra SA, Gabriele M et al, Continuation treatment of delusional depression in older adults, *Am J Geriatr Psychiatry* (2001) **9**:415–22.

Meyers BS, Peasley-Miklus C, Gabriele M et al, NIMH severe depression trial: background and design choices. In: *Syllabus and Proceedings Summary, American Psychiatric Association 2004 Annual Meeting* (American Psychiatric Association: Arlington, VA, 2004) 193–4.

Muller-Siecheneder F, Muller MJ, Hillert A et al, Risperidone versus haloperidol and amitriptyline in the treatment of patients with a combined psychotic and depressive syndrome, *J Clin Psychopharmacol* (1998) **18**:111–20.

Mulsant BH, Rosen J, Thornton JE, Zubenko JS, A prospective naturalistic study of electroconvulsive therapy in late-life depression, *J Geriatr Psychiatry Neurol* (1991) **4**:3–12.

Mulsant BH, Sweet BA, Rosen J et al, A randomized double-blind comparison of nortriptyline plus perphenazine vs. nortriptyline plus placebo in the treatment of psychotic depression in late life, *J Clin Psychiatry* (2001) **62**:597–604.

Murphy E, The prognosis of depression in old age, *Br J Psychiatry* (1983) **142**:111–19.

Nelson JC, Davis JM, DST studies in psychotic depression: a meta-analysis, *Am J Psychiatry* (1997) **154**:1497–503.

Nelson WH, Khan A, Orr WW, Delusional depression: phenomenology, neuroendocrine function, and tricyclic antidepressant response, *J Affect Disord* (1984) **6**:297–306.

Ohayon MM, Schatzberg AF, Prevalence of depressive episodes with psychotic features in the general population, *Am J Psychiatry* (2002) **159**:1855–61.

Pande A, Grunhaus L, Hasket R, Greden JF, Electroconvulsive therapy in delusional and nondelusional depressive disorder, *J Affect Disord* (1990) **19**:215–9.

Parker G, Classifying depression: should lost paradigms be regained, *Am J Psychiatry* (2000) **157**:1195–203.

Parker G, Snowdon J, Parker K, Modelling late-life depression, *Int J Geriatr Psychiatry* (2003) **18**:1102–9.

Parker G, Roy K, Hadzi-Pavlovic D, Pedic F, Psychotic (delusional) depression: a meta-analysis of physical treatments, *J Affect Disord* (1992) **24**:17–24.

Post F, The management and nature of depressive illness in late life: a follow-through study, *Br J Psychiatry* (1972) **21**:393–404.

Roose SP, Glassman AH, Walsh BT et al, Depression, delusions and suicide, *Am J Psychiatry* (1983) **140**:1159–62.

Rothschild AJ, Challenges in the treatment of depression with psychotic features, *Biol Psychiatry* (2003) **53**:680–90.

Rothschild AJ, Phillips KA, Selective serotonin reuptake inhibitors and delusional depression, *Am J Psychiatry* (1999) **156**:977–8.

Rothschild AJ, Benes F, Hebben N et al, Relationships between brain CT scan findings and cortisol in psychotic and nonpsychotic depressed patients, *Biol Psychiatry* (1989) **26**:565–75.

Sackeim H, Brain structure in late-life depression. In: Morisha JM, ed, *Advances in Brain Imaging. Review of Psychiatry*, Vol. 20 (American Psychiatric Association: Washington, DC, 2001) 83–122.

Saunders PA, Copeland JRM, Dewey ME et al, The prevalence of dementia, depression and neurosis in later life: the Liverpool MRC-ALPHA study, *Int J Epidemiol* (1993) 22:838–47.

Schatzberg AF, Rothschild AJ, Psychotic (delusional) major depression: should it be included as a distinct syndrome in DSM-IV?, *Am J Psychiatry* (1992) **149**:733–45.

Snowdon J, The prevalence of depression in old age, *Int J Geriatr Psychiatry* (1990) 5:141–4.

Spiker DG, Weiss JC, Dealy RS et al, The pharmacological treatment of delusional depression, *Am J Psychiatry* (1985) **142**:430–6.

Strober M, Carlson G, Bipolar illness in adolescents with major depression: clinical, genetic, and psychopharmacologic predictors in a three- to four-year prospective follow-up investigation, *Arch Gen Psychiatry* (1982) **39**:549–55.

Vythilingam M, Chen J, Bremner JD et al, Psychotic depression and mortality, *Am J Psychiatry* (2003) **160**:574–6.

World Health Organization, *The ICD-10 Classification of Mental and Behavioural Disorders: Diagnostic Criteria for Research* (World Health Organization: Geneva, 1992).

Zanardi R, Franchini L, Gasperini M et al, Double-blind controlled trial of sertraline versus paroxetine in the treatment of delusional depression, *Am J Psychiatry* (1996) **153**:1631–3.

Zanardi R, Franchini L, Serretti A et al, Venlafaxine versus fluvoxamine in the treatment of delusional depression, *J Clin Psychiatry* (2000) **61**:26–9.

chapter 13

Psychosis in affective disorders – bipolar disorder

Martha Sajatovic and Laszlo Gyulai

Introduction

The Depression and Bipolar Support Alliance recently held a Consensus Development Panel to evaluate progress made during the past decade in late-life affective disorders, and to identify unmet needs in health care delivery and research. This panel, composed of multidisciplinary experts in a variety of relevant fields, concluded that despite encouraging and important advances made in safe and effective treatments, mood disorders remain a significant health care issue for the elderly (Charney et al, 2003). Older adults with affective disorders frequently experience disability and functional decline, reduced quality of life, increased health services use, and caregiver burden, as well as higher mortality rates compared with older individuals without affective disorders (Bartels et al, 2000; Angst et al, 2002; Charney et al, 2003).

In the area of late-life bipolar disorder there is a strong need for better understanding of late-life bipolar phenomenology and disease outcome and identification of optimal treatments based upon controlled trial methodologies, as well as a need for delivery of health care services that take into account the many complexities of treatment in late-life bipolar illness such as medical co-morbidity, care access difficulties, and polypharmacy (Cassano et al, 2000; Almeida and Fenner, 2002; Sajatovic 2002a; Moorhead and Young, 2003; Sajatovic et al, 2004c). Due to a scarcity of published, evidence-based data, current clinical treatment guidelines for bipolar disorder address late-life bipolar disorder only in fairly general terms (Van Gerpen et al, 1999;

Goodwin et al, 2003; American Psychiatric Association, 2002). The majority of clinical treatment recommendations are based on retrospective findings, small studies, open trials, and extrapolations from mixed populations with bipolar disorder (Sajatovic et al, 2003; Young et al, 2004). However, increasing sophistication in the diagnosis and treatment of bipolar disorder in mixed populations (Hirschfeld et al, 2003), aging trends (Krishnan, 2002), and a greater appreciation of the burdens and costs associated with late-life mood disorders (Bartels et al, 2000; Charney et al, 2003; Shulman et al, 2003) have enhanced interest in late-life bipolar disorder. This chapter will overview key issues in late-life bipolar disorder including prevalence and illness presentation, secondary mania, health services use in late-life bipolar illness, treatment complexities, and geriatric psychopharmacology as it relates to late-life bipolar disorder. The chapter concludes with a summary of needed future research in late-life bipolar disorder.

Prevalence, presentation and prognosis

Prevalence of bipolar disorder ranges from 0.1% to 0.4% among older adults over the age of 65 (Van Gerpen et al, 1999). However, this relatively low figure may reflect an under-recognition of late-life bipolar illness, as it is known that elderly individuals may under-report psychiatric symptoms and may be treated in nonspecialty care settings such as nursing homes where psychiatric illness may go undetected by typical survey or assessment methods (McDonald, 2000). In clinical samples, numbers of older adults with bipolar disorder are highly dependent on sample type and sample selection. A recent analysis of a large Psychosis Registry within the United States Veterans Health Administration (VHA) noted that nearly 25% of individuals with bipolar disorder ($n = 16,330$) are age 60 or older, and over 10% are age 70 or older ($n = 8148$) (Sajatovic et al, 2004c). On geriatric psychiatry inpatient units, it has been reported that 5–12% of admissions are patients with bipolar disorder (Yassa et al, 1988; Van Gerpen et al, 1999).

Bipolar disorder in later life may be illness which began in early adulthood and has persisted chronically into late life or, alternatively, may be illness of relatively new onset. While the majority of individuals with bipolar disorder have illness onset in young adulthood, it has been reported that approximately 10% of all patients with bipolar disorder develop new onset illness after the age of 50 (Yassa et al, 1988; Van Gerpen et al, 1999; Almeida and Fenner, 2002). It is possible that growing awareness of bipolar disorder in the community may be driving increased diagnosis of illness and subsequent increased utilization of mental health services for bipolar illness in later life. Almeida and Fenner (2002) recently reported on a mental health services use registry involving over 6000 individuals whose primary or secondary clinical diagnosis was bipolar disorder. In this report, the relative frequency of late-onset bipolar disorder increased from 1% in 1980 to 11% in 1998.

Late-onset bipolar disorder, referring to illness which first manifests late in older adulthood has received relatively limited study (Goodwin and Jamison, 1990; Tohen et al, 1994; Wylie et al, 1999; Cassidy and Carroll, 2002; Moorhead and Young, 2003) and a standardized definition of criteria for late-onset illness has still not been clearly determined (Sajatovic, 2002b). Most, but not all research studies refer to 'late-onset' bipolar disorder as illness which first manifests at age 50 or older. A consistent thread in the available data on late-onset bipolar disorder is the presence of underlying neurological/medical illness among individuals with apparently late-onset mania (Goodwin and Jamison, 1990; Tohen et al, 1994; Shulman, 1997; Cassidy and Carroll, 2002). Goodwin and Jamison (1990) noted that individuals with late-onset bipolar disorder are less likely to have a positive family history of mood disorders compared with individuals with earlier-onset bipolar disorder. Cassidy and Carroll (2002) reported that late-onset mania is associated with elevated vascular risks/vascular disorder including smoking, hypertension, diabetes, coronary artery disease, and atrial fibrillation. It has been suggested that individuals with late-onset mania have a symptom presentation that is milder than that seen in younger individuals (Cassano et al, 2000). However, irritability may be a particular component among the observed behavioral characteristics (James, 1977). In some individuals there may be mixed manic dysphoric or agitated states, psychosis (Wylie et al, 1999) and clinical presentation may mimic a dementia.

There is a relative paucity of published information on prognosis and course of late-life bipolar disorder. Earlier reports suggest more treatment resistance (Van Gerpen et al, 1999) and higher mortality rates (James, 1977; Dhingra and Rabins, 1991; Shulman and Tohen, 1994; Tohen et al, 1994). Angst and colleagues (2003) recently reported on life-long recurrence risk of bipolar I and bipolar II illness. In this report, which evaluated 160 individuals with bipolar I disorder and 60 individuals with bipolar II disorder, cumulative intensity curves for the transition from states of remission to new episodes remained linear over 30–40 years after onset, indicating a constant risk of recurrence over the lifespan up to the age of 70 or more (Angst et al, 2003). Long-term, prospective studies on individuals with bipolar disorder suggest that mortality is elevated due to suicide and cardiovascular disease (Angst et al, 2002). A notable and concerning finding is the persistent high suicide risk over decades for some individuals with bipolar disorder (Angst, et al, 2002).

Secondary mania and bipolar disorder with central nervous system (CNS) co-morbidity

Secondary mania, that is mania causally related to medical or neurologic disease, comprises a heterogeneous group, with etiologies including stroke, traumatic head injury, tumors, and seizures (Shulman, 1997; Van Gerpen et al, 1999; Evans, 2000). The CNS structures that are most often involved are in the right hemisphere of the brain, and include the basal ganglia, thalamic nuclei, orbitofrontal cortex, baso-temporal cortex, and basal forebrain region (Shulman, 1997). Shulman (1997) reported that damage in the right baso-temporal, orbito-frontal cortices, thalamic or caudate nuclei are present in 70.6% of patients with secondary mania. In a study that included elderly patients, Gyulai et al (1997) found an asymmetric distribution of blood flow between the right and left anterior temporal lobes in patients with rapid cycling bipolar disorder.

Bipolar disorder in the elderly is frequently (17–43% of cases) associated with demonstrable cerebral organic disorder (Van Gerpen et al, 1999). A retrospective cohort study found that 72% of patients with late-onset mania had neurological disorders and 42.9% had psychosis (Tohen et al, 1994). Stone (1989) reported that 23.9% of 99 hospitalized elderly manic patients had cerebral organic impairment as indicated by short-term memory loss, disorientation or confusion. In this report by Stone (1989) specific neurological illnesses, such as Parkinson's disease, cerebrovascular accident (CVA) or seizures, were present in 8.7% of the patients. However, only three (3.3%) of these patients had no previous affective illness, and thus appeared to have true secondary mania. Shulman and Post (1980) found that of 67 elderly bipolar patients, 23.9% had co-morbid cerebral-organic disorders, although the etiological significance of these for secondary bipolar disorder could not be established. Finally, Snowdon (1991) found that 17.3% of 75 elderly patients with bipolar disorder had cerebral/neurological illnesses before the onset of mania.

As noted previously, there may be overlap between late-onset bipolar disorder and mania of secondary origin. Silent cerebral infarctions, diagnosed by magnetic resonance imaging (MRI), are associated with approximately 50% of late-onset (mania first occurring after the age of 50) mania cases, and occur in 20% of manic patients who are age 60 or older (Kobayashi et al, 1991; Fujikawa et al, 1995). In elderly manic patients, increasing age is associated with more pronounced subcortical MRI hyperintensities especially in the frontal lobes (McDonald, 1991).

There have been conflicting results regarding whether dementia predisposes to bipolar disorder (Spicer et al, 1973; Shulman and Post, 1980; Cowdry and Goodwin, 1981; Burns et al, 1990; Dhingra and Rabins, 1991; Shulman et al, 1992). Burns et al (1990) and Lyketsos et al (1995) found a 3.5% and 2.2% prevalence of mania in Alzheimer's disease, respectively. Recently, Nilsson et al (2002) showed that patients with dementia are at increased risk of being hospitalized for both mania and depression. Broadhead and Jacoby (1990) found that older patients with bipolar disorder have cortical atrophy, and that both cortical atrophy and ventricular brain ratio (VBR) have a strong positive association with age.

Clinical characteristics of secondary mania in the elderly may differ in a number of aspects compared with 'primary' mania in late life. Selected salient comparative characteristics of primary and secondary mania are shown in Table 13.1. The course of secondary mania is characterized by higher morbidity, mortality, and treatment resistance compared with primary mania (Van Gerpen et al, 1999). Recurrent major depressive episodes most often precede the first episode of mania in late life (Shulman and Post, 1980). Limitations of the literature on secondary mania include the relatively low number of patients, lack of clear data of temporal association between the onset of medical/neurological and psychiatric illness/mania, and the existence of only a few prospective studies.

Health resource use

Published data on health resource utilization patterns among older adults with bipolar disorder support the notion that bipolar disorder does not 'burn out' over time, and that late-life bipolar disorder may be persistent, chronic, and refractory to treatment (Sajatovic et al, 1996; Bartels et al, 2000). Bartels et al (2000) compared mental health service use among elderly patients with bipolar disorder to elderly patients with unipolar depression. In this report older adults with bipolar disorder used nearly four times the total amount of mental health services and were four times more likely to have had a psychiatric hospitalization in the previous six months compared with older

Table 13.1 Comparative features of elderly patients with primary and secondary mania

Features	Primary mania	Secondary mania/co-morbid CNS illness
Age of onset (years), mean (range)	AI: 56.0 (Stone, 1989)* AI: 46.5 (17–73) (Snowdon, 1991)* M: 58.0 (Snowdon, 1991)*	AI: 61.0 (Stone, 1989)* AI: 53 (17–70) (Snowdon, 1991)* M: 63.6 (Snowdon, 1991)*
Gender ratio (female:male)	2.17:1 (Stone, 1989)† 6.28:1 (Shulman and Post, 1980) 2.7:1 (Snowdon, 1991)	0.45:1 (Shulman and Post, 1980) 1.2:1 (Snowdon, 1991)
First episode polarity (%)	Depression: 61%; mania or mixed: 25% (Snowdon, 1991) Depression: 60% (Broadhead and Jacoby, 1990) Depression: 62.7%; mania: 22.4%; mixed: 13.4% (Shulman and Post, 1980)†	Depression: 66%; mania or mixed: 44% (Snowdon, 1991)
Treatment outcome	51% rehospitalized (Stone, 1989)† 72% symptom-free; 16% depressed; 12% (hypo)manic; 32% hospitalized (Dhingra and Rabins, 1991)	Risk of rehospitalization higher (odds ratio 4.6), risk of institutionalization is higher with neurological disorders (odds ratio: 7.7) than without (Shulman, 1992)
Response to lithium	1.1 Rehospitalizations/pt/3.2 years on lithium versus 1.6 rehospitalizations/pt/3.2 years without lithium treatment (NS) (Stone, 1989)†	Poor responders, low dose/serum [Li] ratio, increased probability of lithium neurotoxicity (Himmelhoch et al, 1980)
Family history of affective disorders	32.8% (Stone, 1989)* 48.2% (Snowdon, 1991)* 52% (Shulman et al, 1992)*	9.5% (Stone, 1989)* 15.4% (Snowdon, 1991)* 33% (Shulman et al, 1992)*
CNS/neurological co-morbidity (% patients)	27.7% with early-onset mania (Tohen et al, 1994)	71.4% with late-onset first mania (Tohen et al, 1994) 36% with late-onset mania (Shulman et al, 1992) 17% of all patients (Snowdon, 1991)
Mortality %/years	16%/2 years (Stone, 1989)†	83.3%/4.5 years (Tohen et al, 1994)†

NS, not significant; CNS, central nervous system; AI, affective illness; M, mania; Li, lithium. *Statistical analysis with significance at $p < 0.05$ between primary and secondary bipolar disorder. †Total sample with at least 75% of patients in this illness category (primary or secondary mania).

patients with depression. Additionally, individuals with bipolar disorder had more severe psychiatric symptoms and more impaired community-living skills. Sajatovic et al (2004a) recently reported on a large Veterans Health Administration (VHA) data-base which examined health resource utilization in veterans with bipolar disorder. This report compared health resource use among three groups of veterans with bipolar disorder: 1) those aged 60 and older (*n* = 16,330), 2) those aged 30–59 (*n* = 47,613), and 3) those under age 30 (*n* = 1613). Overall, veterans aged 60 and older were hospitalized at slightly lower rates than younger veterans, but once hospitalized had signifi-cantly longer hospital stays. Veterans aged 60 and older had fairly similar uti-lization of overall outpatient services compared to veterans aged 30–59; however, the younger group had greater utilization of mental health and sub-stance abuse services. It appears that a greater proportion of outpatient serv-ice use by individuals with bipolar disorder aged 60 and older is accounted for by primary care visits. Table 13.2 identifies selected resource utilization differences seen among veterans with bipolar disorder based on age.

Table 13.2 Health resource utilization among veterans with bipolar disorder*

Parameter	Individuals aged 30–59 (n = 47,613)	Individuals aged 60 and older (n = 16,330)	p value
Mean age	47.7 ± SD 7.2	70.2 ± 7.05	. . .
Hospital length of stay (in days)†	60.4 ± 7.4	98.2 ± 215.7	< 0.001
Number of hospitalizations†	6.8 ± 7.4	6.1 ± 6.2	< 0.001
Outpatient service use (total number of all types of visits)††	111.3 ± 146.3	108.5 ± 153.4	< 0.001
Mental health visits‡	53.1 ± 104.2	36.5 ± 102.6	< 0.001
Substance abuse visits	14.8 ± 52.2	3.3 ± 24.7	< 0.001

*From Sajatovic et al, (2004a).

†Hospital inpatient use during Federal Fiscal Year 1998–2000 for patients with bipolar disorder who utilized inpatient services in Federal Fiscal Year 2001.

††Outpatient use during Federal Fiscal Year 1998–2000 for patients with bipolar disorder who used outpatient care in 2001.

‡Mental health care included combined general psychiatry care, post-traumatic stress disorder (PTSD), psychiatric case management/day treatment/vocational clinic and homelessness clinic.

Outcomes of both early- and late-onset bipolar disorder have not been well studied. McDonald and Nemeroff (1996) reported that late-onset mania may be associated with under-recognition of mood symptoms by providers, with resultant increased caregiver burden, functional decline, and possible premature nursing home placement. Unfortunately, resource utilization studies in late-life bipolar disorder have been limited (Sajatovic et al, 2004a) and there are multiple gaps in our understanding of treatment needs and outcome expectations for late-life bipolar disorder.

Treatment complexities

In addition to psychiatric co-morbidity, medical co-morbidity among older adults with bipolar disorder is a particular concern. Sajatovic and colleagues (2003) reported that older adults with bipolar disorder discharged from an inpatient geropsychiatric unit (mean age $67.3 \pm SD$ 10.4 years, $n = 48$) had a mean of 3.7 medical illnesses, including hypertension (69%, $n = 33/48$), diabetes (31.3%, $n = 15/33$), coronary artery disease (25%, $n = 12/48$), arthritis (21%, $n = 10/48$), thyroid disease (17%, $n = 8/48$), and chronic obstructive pulmonary disease (15%, $n = 7/48$). Ruzickova et al (2003) reported that individuals with bipolar disorder and diabetes are likely to be older than individuals without diabetes, and additionally have higher rates of hypertension and higher body mass index. Diabetes co-morbid with bipolar illness is significantly associated with bipolar course chronicity and more disability (Ruzickova et al, 2003). Kessing and Nilsson (2003) noted that patients with bipolar disorder are at greater risk of receiving a diagnosis of dementia than patients with osteoarthritis or diabetes. It is likely that increased medical illness burden contributes to increased utilization of outpatient services for older adults with bipolar disorder compared with younger individuals with bipolar disorder (Sajatovic et al, 2004c). In addition, treatment decisions may be at least partially determined by medical co-morbidity. Electroconvulsive therapy (ECT), the 'gold standard' for the treatment of depression, is still a valid and often optimal intervention for individuals with serious mood disorder and substantial co-existent medical illness. These individuals are likely to be older and require a practitioner with solid clinical knowledge of the fields of medicine and psychiatry (Christopher, 2003)

Polypharmacy, or use of multiple medications, is an additional factor that is likely to complicate treatment and treatment outcomes among older adults with bipolar illness. Surveys of medication use in the elderly suggest an average daily use of approximately seven medications (Cloyd and Locker, 1994). It is known that polypharmacy is independently associated with adverse drug reactions (Onder et al, 2002), and the likelihood of severe drug reactions increases with age (Pollack, 1999). Sajatovic and colleagues (2003) noted that elderly inpatients with bipolar disorder had extensive use of multiple psychotropic medications, with 64% ($n = 16$) of cases on antipsychotic drugs, 72% ($n = 18$) on mood stabilizers, and 44% ($n = 11$) on antidepressant drugs. Finally, in addition to increasing vulnerability to adverse effects, multi-drug regimens are more likely to be associated with poor treatment adherence (Salzman, 1995).

Treatment of late-life bipolar disorder

Bipolar mania

Lithium is still widely used to treat mania in old age (Sajatovic et al, 2004c) and has been used since the discovery of the psychotropic properties of lithium. In spite of its extensive use the evidence for the efficacy of lithium in geriatric mania relies on retrospective, naturalistic studies, case series or extrapolated data from mixed population studies, and no placebo-controlled, randomized trials have been carried out in the geriatric bipolar population (Sajatovic, 2002b; Young et al, 2004). Table 13.3 shows the results of selected acute and maintenance studies relevant to an older population, which involve the use of lithium in bipolar disorder: 30–70% of manic patients benefited from treatment with lithium acutely, but the maintenance efficacy of lithium in the elderly is equivocal. Adjuvant medications were used in most of the studies. There are conflicting data regarding whether older manic patients require lower doses and a lower serum lithium level for efficacious treatment of acute mania than younger populations (Roose et al, 1979; Foster, 1992; Chen et al, 1999). Chen et al (1999) suggested that the elderly benefit from the same serum lithium concentrations utilized in mixed aged adults. However, using a decreased dose of lithium salts is advisable in situations of lower renal clearance of lithium, cardiac disease, and treatment with diuretics (Sajatovic, 2002b). Himmelhoch et al (1980) found that elderly patients with cerebral/neurological disease become toxic more easily on routine doses of lithium, and Foster (1992) has noted that 11–23% of geriatric patients become acutely toxic on lithium.

Prescriptions of divalproex for the treatment of bipolar disorder in the elderly are increasing (Shulman et al, 2003), but there are no controlled studies examining the efficacy of valproate in the treatment of acute mania. There are

Table 13.3 Selected studies relevant to the use of *lithium* in late-life bipolar disorder

Study	Design	n	Age (years) Mean ± SD or range	Diagnosis	Concentration (mEq/l) (range)	Duration	Co-medications	Outcome	Correlates of response
Himmelhoch et al, 1980	Retrospective, open-label, acute	81	63.3 ± 6.9	BP I: 74 BP II: 7	ND	3–8 weeks acute	...	69% improved on a 6-point scale	CNS illness (demetiform syndrome or extrapyramidal dysfunction or drug abuse impairs response
Chen et al, 1999	Retrospective, open-label, acute	30	69.4 ± 8.2	BP, manic or mixed, 67% psychotic	0.30–1.30	2.3 weeks acute	Antipsychotics, benzodiazepines	67% improved	Serum [Li] (87% of patients improved on [Li]$_{ss}$] ≥ 0.8)
van der Velde, 1970	Prospective, open-label with acute and maintenance phase	12	67.0 ± 4.1	BP, manic	0.60–2.00	2 weeks acute and 36 weeks maintenance	Phenothiazines depending on clinical need	4 (33%) improved initially, 1 (0.8%) sustained recovery	Older age predicts worse acute and long-term response
Murray et al, 1983	Prospective maintenance	121	20–79, 25 patients were 60–79	BP	0.65–0.8	24 weeks	Various antimanic medications, antidepressants, hypnotic/sedatives as needed	Mania in 6% of the visits; depression in 15% of the visits	Age has a mild negative effect for mania but not for depression

BP, bipolar disorder; ND, no data; Li, lithium.

few studies indicating efficacy of divalproex for geriatric mania. Table 13.4 shows selected relevant studies with respect to older adults, involving the use of valproate in bipolar disorder; 60–90% of manic patients had a favorable response to valproate. There are no maintenance studies in the elderly. Valproate was tolerated well in these studies, with doses ranging from 250 to 2250 mg per day and achieving total valproate concentrations between 25 and 120 μg/ml.

A retrospective study of older patients treated with lithium or divalproex sodium (n = 59) found that 66% of acutely manic patients had psychotic features (Chen et al, 1999). In that same report, approximately 60% of the patients were treated with an antipsychotic medication. Colenda (2002) provided a summary of approaches to management of mania in late life that includes the use of atypical antipsychotics as well as lithium and anti-epilepsy medications. While promising, the evidence for the efficacy of antipsychotic drugs for treating mania in the elderly is based upon anecdotes or small/open studies, and randomized controlled studies are lacking (Sajatovic, 2002b). In studies illustrated in Table 13.4, 67–86% of patients were psychotic at study entry and a combination of classical and atypical antipsychotic medications with valproate and lithium was often used with few major adverse events. Preliminary data indicate that olanzapine, clozapine, and quetiapine can be helpful in the treatment of geriatric mania.

Bipolar depression

There are no systematic studies examining the treatment of geriatric bipolar depression. Lamotrigine (75–100 mg/day) has been shown to be useful as add-on treatment to lithium or divalproex in elderly bipolar depressed patients (Robillard and Conn, 2002). Lamotrigine may also be useful as a maintenance therapy in geriatric bipolar disorder (Sajatovic, in press). Antidepressant medications, particularly the selective serotonin reuptake inhibitor (SSRI) compounds, are widely utilized in clinical settings for geriatric bipolar depression (Sajatovic et al, 2004b). Oshima and Higuchi (1999) noted that although current Food and Drug Administration (FDA)-approved antidepressants appear to be equally effective in older adults with depression, compounds with lower anticholinergic and anti-alpha 1 effects are better tolerated in geriatric patients. Some elderly patients will derive antidepressant effects from lithium as well (Oshima and Higuchi, 1999). Finally, similar to unipolar depression, it is important to consider the role of ECT for treating both manic and depressed phases in the elderly bipolar patient (Thienhaus et al, 1990; Gareri et al, 2000).

Table 13.4 Selected studies relevant to the use of valproate in late-life bipolar disorder

Study	Design	n	Age (years) mean ± SD or (range)	Diagnosis	Concentration (mg/l) mean ± SD or (range)	Duration (weeks)	Co-medications	Outcome	Correlates of outcome
McFarland et al, 1990	Prospective, open-label	7	66.3 ± 6.4	BP, manic or mixed, one patient had psychotic depression	Target: 50–150	4	Antipsychotics, antidepressants, Li, benzodiazepines, thyroid replacement	83.3% of bipolar patients moderately or markedly improved	...
Noaghiul et al, 1998	Retrospective, open-label, acute, inpatient	21	70.5 ± 7.1	BP, manic 86% psychotic	71.9 ± 20.7	1.1–6.7 (median 2)	Antipsychotics, including 5 patients on atypical antipsychotics, 5 patients on Li	90% of patients much or very much improved	Dose of divalproex (+) Baseline Young Mania Rating Scale (−)
Kando et al, 1996	Retrospective, open-label	35	71.3 (63–85)	68.6% BP-I, manic, 31.4% other affective disorder	52.9 ± 21.6	4.7 (range: 0.4–21.4)	Classical antipsychotics, clozapine, antidepressants, Li, benzodiazepines	62% of bipolar patients moderately or markedly improved with adequate trial	None found
Niedermier and Nasrallah, 1998	Retrospective, open-label, acute, inpatient	39	67 (60–86)	16 BP, 7 BP and dementia, 10 dementia, 6 other 71% psychotic	72 (36–111)	>1	Classical and atypical antipsychotics, SSRI antidepressants, Li, benzodiazepines	14/16 (88%) BP responded; 7 (100%) BP and dementia responded	Bipolar diagnosis (+), female (+), age (−), [valproate]$_{ss}$ concentrations (−), fewer psychotic symptoms (+)
Chen et al, 1999	Retrospective, open-label, acute, inpatient	29	71.2 ± 8.2	BP, manic, 67% psychotic	65–90 for 8 patients, 25–64 or 90–130 all others	2.2 ± 1.0	Antipsychotics, benzodiazepines until discharge from hospital	75% of patients with [valproate]$_{ss}$ of 65–90 mg/l improved	Serum [valproate]-[vaproate]$_{ss}$ of 65–90 mg/l correlates with best outcome

BP, bipolar disorder; Li, lithium; SSRI, selective serotonin reuptake inhibitor.

Psychotherapy and psychosocial interventions

Specific contemporary models of psychotherapy, such as cognitive behavioral therapy (CBT), interpersonal psychotherapy (IPT), and family-focused therapy have been demonstrated to be of benefit in the treatment of bipolar disorder (Miklowitz and Frank, 1999; Craighead and Miklowitz, 2000; Frank and Novick, 2001). Psychotherapies that have been reported to be useful with older adults include CBT, IPT, family therapy, and group therapies (Teri and Logsdon, 1992; Scogin and McElreath, 1994; Kodar et al, 1996; Weissman, 1997). In some instances, such as with IPT, standardized therapies have been modified for the elderly (Weissman, 1997). Factors that may be of particular relevance with respect to psychotherapeutic interventions in the elderly include ongoing assessment of suicidality given greater vulnerability to suicide among older male populations (Sachs et al, 2001) and a need for stable and consistent treatment routine in patients who are struggling with symptoms and disability as well as possible emergent medical comorbidity (Frank et al, 1999). Common life-stage issues for older adults include retirement and job loss, loss of societal and financial status, medical illness and loss/change in social supports due to illness or death. Ideally, these factors must be addressed in the context of an effective psychotherapeutic intervention for older adults with bipolar disorder.

Conclusions and future research directions

In the face of changing demographics, it is critical that there is increased knowledge and greater awareness of the clinical presentation, clinical needs, and treatment outcomes of older adults with bipolar disorder. Geriatric bipolar disorder imposes a substantial burden on patients, their families, and increasingly, our health care systems. The bulk of current knowledge is based on extrapolated results from younger populations, an approach that is not likely to lead to a clear picture of bipolar disorder in late life. Important issues such as identification of criteria for late-onset illness, understanding of age-related changes likely to be seen in individuals with bipolar disorder, and data specific to older adults with respect to treatment and symptomatic and functional treatment outcomes remain to be fully addressed. Additional research is needed in order to use evidence-based data for improving health services delivery for older adults with bipolar disorder.

References

Almeida OP, Fenner S, Bipolar disorder: similarities and differences between patients with illness onset before and after 65 years of age, *Int Psychogeriatrics* (2002) 14:311–22.

American Psychiatric Association, Practice guidelines for the treatment of patients with bipolar disorder, revision, *Am J Psychiatry* (2002) 159:1–50.

Angst F, Stassen HH, Clayton PJ, Angst J, Mortality of patients with mood disorders: follow-up over 34–38 years, *J Affective Disord* (2002) 68: 167–81.

Angst J, Gamma A, Sellaro R et al, Recurrence of bipolar disorders and major depression. A life-long perspective, *Eur Arch Psychiatry Clin Neurosci* (2003) 253:236–40.

Bartels SJ, Forster B, Miles KM et al, Mental health service use by elderly patients with bipolar disorder and unipolar major depression, *Am J Geriatr Psychiatry* (2000) 8:160–6.

Broadhead J, Jacoby R, Mania in old age: a first prospective study, *Int J Geriatr Psychiatry* (1990) 59 (suppl 1):S69–S79.

Burns A, Jacoby R, Levy R, Psychiatric phenomena in Alzheimer disease. II: Disorders of mood, *Br J Psychiatry* (1990) 157:81–6.

Cassano GB, McElroy SL, Brady K et al, Current issues in the identification and management of bipolar spectrum disorders in 'Special populations', *J Affect Disord* (2000) 59 (suppl 1): S69–S79.

Cassidy F, Carroll BJ, Vascular risk factors in late onset mania, *Psychol Med* (2002) 32:359–362.

Charney DS, Reynolds CF, Lebowitz BL et al, Depression and bipolar support alliance consensus statement on the unmet needs in diagnosis and treatment of mood disorders in late life, *Arch Gen Psychiatry* (2003) 60:664–72.

Chen ST, Altshuler LL, Melnyk KA et al, Efficacy of lithium vs. valproate in the treatment of mania in the elderly: a retrospective study, *J Clin Psychiatry* (1999) 60:181–6.

Christopher EJ, Electroconvulsive therapy in the medically ill, *Curr Psychiatry Rep* (2003) 5: 225–30.

Cloyd JC, Locker TE, Antiepileptic drugs in the elderly: pharmacoepidemiology and pharmacokinetics, *Arch Family Med* (1994) 3:589–98.

Colenda CC, Mania in late life: the challenges of treating older adults, *Geriatrics* (2002) 57:50–4.

Cowdry RW, Goodwin FK, Dementia in bipolar illness: diagnosis and response to lithium, *Am J Psychiatry* (1981) 138:1118–19.

Craighead WE, Miklowitz DJ, Psychosocial interventions for bipolar disorder, *J Clin Psychiatry* (2000) 61 (suppl 13):58–64.

Dhingra U, Rabins PV, Mania in the elderly: a 5–7 year follow-up, *J Am Geriatr Soc* (1991) 39:581–3.

Evans D, Bipolar disorder: diagnostic challenges and treatment considerations, *J Clin Psychiatry* (2000) 61 (suppl 13):26–31.

Foster JR, Use of lithium in elderly psychiatric patients: a review of the literature, *Lithium* (1992) 3:77–93.

Frank E, Novick D, Progress in the psychotherapy of mood disorders: studies from the Western Psychiatric Institute and Clinic, *Epidemiol Psychiatr Soc* (2001) 10:245–52.

Frank E, Swartz HA, Mallinger AG et al, Adjunctive psychotherapy for bipolar disorder: effects of changing treatment modality, *J Abnormal Psychol* (1999) 108:579–87.

Fujikawa T, Yamakawi S, Touhaouda Y, Silent cerebral infarction in patients with late-onset mania, *Stroke* (1995) 26:946–9.

Gareri P, Falconi U, De Fazio P, De Sarro G, Conventional and new antidepressant drugs in the elderly, *Prog Neurobiol* (2000) 61:353–96.

Goodwin FK, Jamison KR, *Manic Depressive Illness* (Oxford University Press: Oxford, 1990).

Goodwin GM, Consensus Group for the British Association for Psychopharmacology. Evidence-based guidelines for treating bipolar disorder: recommendations from the British Association for Psychopharmacology, *J Psychopharmacol* (2003) **17**:149–73.

Gyulai L, Alavi A, Broich K et al, I-123 iofetamine single-photon computed emission tomography in rapid cycling bipolar disorder: a clinical study, *Biol Psychiatry* (1997) **41**:152–61.

Himmelhoch JM, Neil JF, May SJ et al, Age, dementia, dyskinesias, and lithium response, *Am J Psychiatry* (1980) **137**:941–5.

Hirschfeld RM, Calabrese JR, Weissman MM et al, Screening for bipolar disorder in the community, *J Clin Psychiatry* (2003) **64**:53–9.

James NM, Early and late-onset bipolar affective disorder, *Arch Gen Psychiatry* (1977) **34**:715–17.

Kando JC, Tohen M, Castillo J, Zarate CA Jr, The use of valproate in an elderly population with affective symptoms, *J Clin Psychiatry* (1996) **57**:238–40.

Kessing LV, Nilsson FM, Increased risk of developing dementia in patients with major affective disorders compared to patients with other medical illnesses, *J Affect Disord* (2003) **73**:261–9.

Kobayashi S, Okada K, Yamashita K, Incidence of silent lacunar lesion in normal adults and its relation to cerebral blood flow and risk factors, *Stroke* (1991) **22**:1379–83.

Kodar K, Brodaty H, Anatey K, Cognitive therapy for depression in the elderly, *Int J Geriatr Psychol* (1996) **11**:97.

Krishnan KRR, Biological risk factors in late life depression, *Biol Psychiatry* (2002) **52**:185–92.

Lyketsos CG, Corazzini K, Steele C, Mania in Alzheimer's disease, *J Neuropsychiatry Clin Neurosci* (1995) **7**:350–2.

McDonald WM, Epidemiology, etiology, and treatment of geriatric mania, *J Clin Psychiatry* (2000) **61** (Suppl 13): 3–11.

McDonald WM, Krishnan KR, Doraiswamy PM et al, Occurence of subcortical hyperintensities in elderly subjects with mania, *Psychiatry Research* (1991) **40**:212–20.

McDonald WM, Nemeroff CB, The diagnosis and treatment of mania in the elderly, *Bull Menninger Clin* (1996) **60**:175–337.

McFarland BH, Miller MR, Straumfjord AA, Valproate use in the older manic patient, *J Clin Psychiatry* (1990) **51**:479–81.

Miklowitz DJ, Frank E, New psychotherapies for bipolar disorder. In: Goldberg JF, Harrow M, eds, *Bipolar Disorders: Clinical Course and Outcome* (American Psychiatric Association: Washington, DC, 1999) 57–84.

Moorhead SRJ, Young AH, Evidence for a late onset bipolar-I disorder sub-group from 50 years, *J Affect Disord* (2003) **73**:271–7.

Murray N, Hopwood S, Balfour DJ et al, The influence of age on lithium efficacy and side-effects in out-patients, *Psychol Med* (1983) **13**:53–60.

Niedermier JA, Nasrallah HA, Clinical correlates of response to valproate in geriatric inpatients, *Ann Clin Psychiatry* (1998) **10**:165–8.

Nilsson FM, Kesing LV, Sornsen RM et al, Enduring increased risk of developing depression and mania in patients with dementia, *J Neurol Neurosurg Psychiatry* (2002) **73**:40–4.

Noaghiul S, Narayan M, Nelson JC, Divalproex treatment of mania in elderly patients, *Am J Geriatr Psychiatry* (1998) **6**:257–62.

Onder G, Pedone C, Landi F et al, Adverse drug reactions as cause of hospital admissions: results from the Italian Group of Pharmacoepidemiology in the Elderly (GIFA), *J Am Geriatr Soc* (2002) **50**:1962–8.

Oshima A, Higuchi T, Treatment guidelines for geriatric mood disorders, *Psychiatry Clin Neurosci* (1999) **53** (Suppl):S55–S59.

Pollack BG, Adverse drug reactions of antidepressants in elderly patients, *J Clin Psychiatry* (1999) **6** (Suppl 20):4–8.

Robillard M, Conn DK, Lamotrigine use in geriatric patients with bipolar depression, *Can J Psychiatry* (2002) **47**:767–70.

Roose SP, Bone S, Haidorfer C et al, Lithium treatment in older patients, *Am J Psychiatry* (1979) **136**:843–4.

Ruzickova M, Slaney C, Garnham J, Alda M, Clinical features of bipolar disorder with and without comorbid diabetes mellitus, *Can J Psychiatry* (2003) **48**:458–61.

Sachs GS, Yan LJ, Swan AC, Allen MH, Integration of suicide prevention into outpatient management of bipolar disorder, *J Clin Psychiatry* (2001) **62** (Suppl 25):3–11.

Sajatovic M, Popli A, Semple W, Health resource utilization over a ten year period by geriatric veterans with schizophrenia and bipolar disorder, *Psychiatr Serv* (1996) **47**:961–5.

Sajatovic M, Aging-related issues in bipolar disorder: a health services perspective, *J Geriatr Psychiatry Neurol* (2002a) **15**:128–33.

Sajatovic M, Treatment of bipolar disorder in older adults, *Int J Geriatr Psychiatry* (2002b) **17**:865–73.

Sajatovic M, Bingham CR, Campbell E, Fletcher E, Bipolar disorder in older adults. Poster presented at the *Annual Meeting of the American Psychiatric Association*, San Francisco, CA, USA, May (2003).

Sajatovic M, Blow F, Ignacio R et al, Bipolar disorder in the VA: aging-related modifiers. Presented at the *17th Annual Meeting of the American Association of Geriatric Psychiatry*, Baltimore, MA, February (2004a).

Sajatovic M, Friedman-Hatters S, Saberwhal J, Bingham CR, Clinical characteristics and hospital based resource use among older adults with bipolar disorder, schizophrenia, depression and dementia, *J Geriatr Psychiatry Neurol* (2004b) **17**:3–8.

Sajatovic M, Blow FC, Ignacio RV et al, Age-related modifiers of clinical presentation and health service among veterans with bipolar disorder, *Psychiatr Serv* (2004c) **55**:1014–21.

Sajatovic M, Gyulai L, Calabrese JR et al, The effect of age on maintenance treatment outcomes in bipolar 1 disorder, *Am J Geriatr Psychiatry* (in press).

Salzman C, Medication compliance in the elderly, *J Clin Psychiatry* (1995) **56 (Suppl 1)**: 18–22.

Scogin F, McElreath L, Efficacy of psychosocial treatments for geriatric depression: a quantitative review, *J Consult Clin Psychol* (1994) **62**:69–71.

Shulman KI, Disinhibition syndromes, secondary mania and bipolar disorder in old age, *J Affect Disord* (1997) **46**:175–82.

Shulman K, Post F, Bipolar affective disorder in old age, *Br J Psychiatry* (1980) **136**: 26–32.

Shulman KI, Tohen M, Unipolar mania reconsidered: evidence from an elderly cohort, *Br J Psychiatry* (1994) **164**:547–9.

Shulman KI, Tohen M, Satlin A et al, Mania compared with unipolar depression in old age, *Am J Psychiatry* (1992) **149**:341–5.

Shulman KI, Rochon P, Suykora K et al, Changing prescription patterns for lithium and valproic acid in old age: shifting practice without evidence, *BMJ* (2003) **326**:960–1.

Snowdon J, Mania in the elderly, *Br J Psychiatry* (1991) **158**:485–90.

Spicer CC, Hare EJ, Slater D, Neurotic and psychotic forms of depressive illness: evidence from age-incidence in a national sample, *Br J Psychiatry* (1973) **123**:535–41.

Stone K, Mania in the elderly, *Br J Psychiatry* (1989) **155**:220–4.

Teri L, Logsdon R, The future of psychotherapy with older adults. Special issue: the future of psychotherapy, *Psychotherapy* (1992): 8.

Thienhaus OJ, Margletta S, Bennet JA, A study of the clinical efficacy of maintenance ECT, *J Clin Psychiatry* (1990) **51**:141–4.

Tohen M, Shulman KI, Satlin A, First-episode mania in late life, *Am J Psychiatry* (1994) **151**:130–2.

Van der Velde CD, Effectiveness of lithium carbonate in the treatment of manic depressive illness, *Am J Psychiatry* (1970) **127**:345–51.

Van Gerpen MW, Johnson JE, Winstead DK, Mania in the geriatric patient population, *Am J Geriatr Psychiatry* (1999) **7**:188–202.

Weissman MM, Interpersonal psychotherapy: current status, *Keio J Med* (1997) **46**:105–10.

Wylie ME, Mulsant BH, Pollock BG et al, Age at onset in geriatric bipolar disorder: effects on clinical presentation and treatment outcomes in an inpatient sample, *Am J Geriatr Psychiatry* (1999) **7**:77–83.

Yassa R, Nair NPV, Iskandar H, Late-onset bipolar disorder, *Psychiatr Clin North Am* (1988) **11**:1171–31.

Young RC, Falk NR, Age, manic psychopathology and treatment response, *Int J Geriatr Psychiatry* (1989) 4.

Young RC, Gyulai L, Mulsant B et al, Pharmacotherapy of bipolar disorder in old age: review and recommendations, *Am J Geriatr Psychiatry* (2004) **12**:342–57.

chapter 14

Psychotic symptoms in dementia

Simon Douglas and Clive Ballard

Introduction

This chapter will briefly summarize key issues related to the nature of psychotic symptoms in people with dementia. This will provide an overview of the definition and measurement of psychosis in dementia, along with an exploration of the incidence and prevalence in Alzheimer's disease (AD) and other different types of dementia, before an examination of current treatment strategies.

Classification of psychosis

Within the context of dementia, Burns et al (1990) classified psychosis into three main categories: delusions, hallucinations, and delusional misidentification. This theoretical classification, detailed further below, is supported by empirical evidence from a principal components analysis of a detailed list of individual symptoms (Ballard et al, 1995).

- **Delusions** – defined as false, unshakeable ideas or beliefs that are held with conviction and subjective certainty. In order to avoid confusion with confabulation of delirium these must be expressed on at least two occasions and more than one week apart.
- **Hallucinations** – described as perceptions in the absence of a stimulus, need to be directly reported either by the patient or indirectly through an informant to be classified as a psychotic presentation and may not be inferred from observed behaviors.
- **Delusional misidentification** – includes: Capgras syndrome; delusional misidentification of visual (television or photographic) images;

delusional misidentification of mirror images; and the 'phantom boarder' delusion.

Although broadly speaking hallucinations, delusions, and delusional misidentification also occur in functional psychoses, there are important differences. Two of the predominant forms of delusional misidentification in dementia, misidentification of mirror images and misidentification of television images are, for example, exclusively seen in organic disorders (Ballard et al, 2001a). In addition, the most common forms of hallucinations are visual, in contrast to functional psychosis where auditory hallucinations predominate. Diagnosing delusions in the presence of dementia can also be difficult. The majority of delusional beliefs are simple, and the complex elaborate delusional symptoms seen in functional psychosis are extremely rare, and are confined to a small number of people in the early stages of the dementia process (Burns et al, 1990). The crux of the issue is to be able to distinguish people who make confabulations or assumptions which can be entirely explained as a result of impairments in higher cognitive functions, from those who are experiencing delusions.

Assessment tools

Psychotic symptoms can be difficult to identify due to the informant's tendency to under-report individual symptoms. It is therefore useful to utilize structured assessment methods, which in studies have accounted for a doubling of frequency of identified symptoms (Ballard et al, 1995). There is a wide range of assessment tools available and they are often brief and suitable for use by a range of health professionals. Among the more widely used and well validated are the BEHAVE-AD (Reisberg et al, 1987) and the Neuropsychiatric Inventory (NPI; Cummings et al, 1994) which take 15–20 minutes to administer, with the NPI having the advantage of a more comprehensive list of psychotic symptoms together with a section rating carer distress. Other studies have utilized operationalized diagnostic criteria such as those of Burns et al (1990), DSM-lllR or DSM-lV (American Psychiatric Association, 1987, 1994), either as the main evaluation tool or in combination with a standardized schedule such as CERAD (Tariot, 1996).

Impact of psychotic symptoms

Psychotic symptoms in dementia can be unpleasant for the patient, with a third of people experiencing these symptoms feeling marked distress (Gilley et al, 1991; Ballard et al, 1995). It has also been observed that psychosis often occurs in conjunction with behavioral disturbances such as aggression or agitation (Rockwell et al, 1994). Dementia patients with psychosis, particularly those experiencing visual hallucinations, have a two- to three-fold accelerated rate of cognitive decline (Chui et al, 1994; Paulsen et al, 2000).

Prevalence, incidence and resolution

Over the course of the illness the cumulative prevalence of psychosis has been put at a rate probably exceeding 80% (Allen and Burns, 1995; Ballard et al, 1997) with a mean prevalence of 44% in clinical samples (hallucinations, overall 21% [auditory 7%, visual 14%], delusions 32%, delusional misidentification 30%). Table 14.1 examines prospective studies utilizing standardized methodology which indicate the cross-sectional prevalence rates of psychosis in a variety of settings from a meta-analysis of the literature in 2001 (Ballard et al, 2001a). There is a paucity of reports from nursing homes (Cohen et al, 1998), although a study has confirmed that psychotic symptoms are evident in more than 20% of nursing home residents with dementia (Margallo-Lana et al, 2001). The lack of nursing home studies is rather a paradox given the reported association (Steele et al, 1990; Haupt et al, 1996) between psychotic symptoms and admission to care facilities.

Annual incidence rates for psychosis range from 1–5% to 46% (Ballard et al, 2001a). Fewer studies have investigated the annual incidence of delusions (range 30–47%) or hallucinations (range 10–20%), although the findings are more consistent (McShane et al, 1995, 1996; Ballard et al, 1997).

Ballard et al (1997, 1998) and McShane et al (1995) reported annual resolution rates of 43–65%, with approximately 50% of symptoms spontaneously resolving over three months; an observation consistent with the extremely high placebo response rates in treatment studies (Schneider et al, 1990).

Clinical associations

Whilst both visual hallucinations and delusions are relatively uncommon amongst people with mild AD (Ballard et al, 1999), the prevalence of

Table 14.1 Prevalence of psychotic symptoms in people with dementia: a summary of standardized studies

Study and year	n	Diagnosis	Delusion prevalence	Hallucination prevalence	Associations reported			
					Auditory hallucination prevalence	Visual hallucination prevalence	General psychosis prevalence	Delusional misidentification prevalence
a) Hospital settings								
Hirono et al, 1998	228	AD	52%	11%	6%	3%	52%	
Gilley et al, 1997	270	AD	47%	41%				
Ballard et al, 1995	124	AD, DLB and VaD	48%		13%	35%	67%	29%
Binetti et al, 1995	99	AD and VaD	24%					11%
Burns et al, 1990	178	AD	16%		10%	13%		
Cooper et al, 1990	677	AD	26%	17%				
Devanand et al, 1992	91	AD			1%	4%		
Sultzer et al, 1993	56	AD and VaD					36%	
Ballard et al, 1991	66	AD	29%	22%				
Ballinger et al, 1982	100			34%				
Jost and Grossberg 1996	100	AD					45%	
Ballard et al, 1997	87						47%	
Mega et al, 1996	50	AD	22%	10%				
Haupt et al, 1996	78	AD	33%	15%	4%	14%		
Cummings et al, 1987	45	AD and VaD	33%	16%	4%	20%		
Mortimer et al, 1992	65	AD	28%					
Holroyd and Sheldon-Keller 1995	98	AD				18%		
Jeste et al, 1992	107	AD	35%		1.9%	12%		
Flynn et al, 1991	33	AD and VaD					69%	
McShane et al, 1995	41	AD				32%		
Migliorelli et al, 1995	103	AD					37%	
Förstl et al, 1994	56		16%	23%	13%	18%		
Chui et al, 1994	135	AD	12%	13%				25%

Study	n	Diagnosis						
Mean			31% (n=686)	21% (n=371)	9% (n=62)	14% (n=144)	44% (n=167)	30% (n=97)
b) Nursing homes								
Morriss et al, 1990	84	AD and VaD	35%				39%	
Rovner et al, 1986	50	AD and VaD					13%	
Chandler and Chandler, 1988	65	AD and VaD						
Mean			35% (n=29)				24% (n=28)	
c) Community								
Hope et al, 1997	97	AD and VaD		29%	17%	19%	37%	
Skoog, 1993	147	AD and VaD	5%				14%	
Gilley et al, 1991	230	AD		29%	19%	19%		11%
Mean			5% (n=8)	29% (n=67)	19% (n=39)	19% (n=44)	23% (n=57)	11% (n=26)
d) Research clinics								
Lopez et al, 1996	40	AD	33%	34%	5%	15%	43%	34%
Drevets and Rabin, 1989	82	AD	43%	24%	16%	32%	27%	30%
Förstl et al, 1993	50	AD	44%	31%	10%	19%	47%	23%
Deutsch et al, 1991	181	AD	34%	18%	16%	22%	15%	
Rosen and Zubenko, 1991	32	AD	38%	76%	6%	15%		
Patterson et al, 1990	34	AD		25%	24%	53%		
Lopez et al, 1991	113	AD	71%		10%	15%	15%	
Rubin et al, 1988	110	AD					56%	
Zubenko et al, 1991	27	AD					48%	
Mean			49% (n=219)	39% (n=190)	13% (n=73)	26% (n=145)	36% (n=146)	28% (n=96)

AD, Alzheimer's disease; DLB, dementia with Lewy bodies; VaD, vascular dementia.

delusions appears to peak in people with AD of moderate severity, whereas visual hallucinations are even more prevalent among those with severe dementia. This perhaps indicates that a certain level of cognitive processing may be necessary in order to generate a delusional belief.

Impaired visual acuity has been identified as a consistent positive association of visual hallucinations (McShane et al, 1995). Although this requires further study, it suggests the possibility that impairments at a variety of levels of the visual pathway may predispose to visual hallucinations in people with dementia. There also appears to be an association between extrapyramidal symptoms and risk of psychosis (Caligiuri et al, 2003).

Biological and experimental correlates of psychosis

Work in this area is at a preliminary stage and the literature is very inconsistent; however, it does appear that delusions and hallucinations may have a different biological basis. Several groups have reported that basal ganglia calcification may be important in the genesis of delusions in some patients (Burns et al, 1990), possibly through 'deficient sensory gating' mechanisms. Förstl et al (1994) suggested that patients with delusional misidentification and those with hallucinations had significantly higher neuron numbers in the parahippocampal gyrus, but lower cell counts in the dorsal raphe nucleus; while patients presenting with delusions had lower neuronal counts in the hippocampus (CA1). Farber et al (2000) reported a significant association between psychosis and the overall severity of neurofibrillary tangles in AD patients, although a subsequent study was unable to confirm this observation (Sweet et al, 2000). A number of reports have highlighted potential associations between various genetic polymorphisms of 5-hydroxytryptamine (5-HT) and dopaminergic receptors and psychosis in AD (Holmes et al, 2001; Nacmias et al, 2001), although most are so far unconfirmed. Parallel studies investigating visual hallucinations in dementia with Lewy bodies (DLB) have indicated an association with cholinergic loss and relative preservation of 5-HT in the temporal cortex (Perry et al, 1993), particularly in the visual association areas. Zubenko et al (1991) reported a link between psychotic symptoms and a reduction of 5-HT, with relative preservation of noradrenaline, but did not identify any associations with dopaminergic parameters. Two recent studies, one focusing on DLB and one focusing on AD, have both demonstrated an association between delusions and altered muscarinic receptor binding (Ballard et al, 2000; Lai et al, 2001).

Psychosis in other common late-onset dementias

Retrospective studies of neuropathologically confirmed cases suggest that visual hallucinations are a key diagnostic feature of DLB, with a prevalence rate of 60% in psychiatric samples and 20% in cohorts from neurology settings (Ballard et al, 1996). DLB patients are more likely to experience accompanying auditory hallucinations (Ballard et al, 1996, 1999), experience their hallucinations more frequently during an average week, are more distressed by their psychosis (Ballard et al, 1995), and experience greater persistence of their psychotic symptoms, especially visual hallucinations (Ballard et al, 1998). The persistence and severity of the symptoms are a particular problem given the limited treatment options, because of the severe neuroleptic sensitivity reactions experienced by many DLB patients (McKeith et al, 1992).

Psychosis in vascular dementia (VaD) has received far less attention; however, a number of small clinical studies have examined rates. The mean prevalence of psychosis is 37% with few differences from AD (Ballard et al, 2001b), although one recent large community study has suggested a reduced frequency of psychosis in VaD compared with AD (Lyketsos et al, 2000). Associations have not been studied, but the focal nature of lesions in VaD may offer important information regarding the regions of interest.

Treatment of psychotic symptoms in dementia

As the natural course of psychosis in AD is to improve, and placebo response rates are extremely high in clinical trials, it is very difficult to infer a great deal from studies other than double-blind placebo-controlled clinical trials. The majority of such studies have evaluated the impact of treatment upon 'generic' behavioral and psychiatric symptoms, although some have included a secondary evaluation of psychosis. Other studies examining the impact of cholinesterase inhibitors on cognition and global performance have measured behavioral and psychiatric symptoms as additional outcome measures, although in most of these latter studies few patients have clinically significant noncognitive symptoms and hence the results are difficult to interpret.

Psychosis has been measured as a secondary outcome measure in several clinical neuroleptic trials, with some evidence of modest but clinically significant benefit with risperidone and olanzapine (Katz et al, 1999; Street et al, 2000; Brodaty et al, 2003). However, recent concerns regarding an increased risk of cerebrovascular adverse events with these two agents (Committee on Safety of Medicines, 2004) limits their potential clinical utility and there are very limited data specifically about the treatment of psychosis from studies utilizing other neuroleptics.

A placebo-controlled trial of the cholinesterase inhibitor rivastigmine in DLB (McKeith et al, 2000) indicated a significant overall effect on neuropsychiatric symptoms, although no sub-analyses were undertaken examining psychosis specifically. Other trials of cholinesterase inhibitors have focused predominantly on cognitive outcome in patients with low levels of psychiatric symptoms. Although there is encouraging preliminary evidence of some effect on overall 'behavioral' scores (Birks and Harvey, 2004; Olin and Schneider, 2004), the potential efficacy on clinically significant psychotic symptoms has not been determined. A study of the muscarinic agonist xanomeline (Mirza et al, 2003) did suggest some benefit with respect to psychotic symptoms, which is consistent with the scientific studies, although poor tolerability limits potential clinical applications.

There are no studies of nonpharmacological interventions focusing on psychosis in dementia, although a recent review highlights some excellent common-sense principles to identify and remove triggers and foci of potential misinterpretation (Cohen-Mansfield, 2003). Correcting any visuospatial impairments may also be helpful (Chapman et al, 1999).

Conclusion

There is a clear and urgent need for specific targeted intervention trials. In the interim, the best clinical advice is probably to avoid pharmacological treatments unless a psychotic symptom is distressing or problematic and to monitor closely. Common sense nonpharmacological interventions are likely to be helpful, but there is no specific evidence. If pharmacological treatments are required, a trial of a cholinesterase inhibitor is probably the preferable first line approach.

References

Allen NHP, Burns A, The non-cognitive features of dementia, *Rev Clin Gerontol* (1995) 5:57–75.

American Psychiatric Association, *Diagnostic and Statistical Manual of Mental Disorders*, 3rd edn (revised) (DSM-III) (American Psychiatric Association: Washington, DC, 1987).

American Psychiatric Association, *Diagnostic and Statistical Manual of Mental Disorders*, 4th edn (DSM-IV) (American Psychiatric Association: Washington, DC, 1994).

Ballard CG, Chithiramohan RN, Bannister C et al, Paranoid features in the elderly with dementia, *Int J Geriatr Psychiatry* (1991) **6**:155–7.

Ballard CG, Saad K, Patel A et al, The prevalence and phenomenology of psychotic symptoms in dementia sufferers, *Int J Geriatr Psychiatry* (1995) **10**:477–85.

Ballard C, Lowery K, Harrison R, McKeith IG, Noncognitive symptoms in Lewy body dementia. In: Perry R, McKeith IG, Perry EK, eds, *Dementia with Lewy Bodies* (Cambridge University Press: Cambridge, 1996).

Ballard C, O'Brien J, Coope B et al, A prospective study of psychotic symptoms in dementia sufferers: psychosis in dementia, *Int Psychogeriatrics* (1997) **9**:57–64.

Ballard CG, O'Brien J, Lowery K et al, A prospective study of dementia with Lewy bodies, *Age Ageing* (1998) **27**:631–6.

Ballard C, Holmes C, McKeith I et al, Psychiatric morbidity in dementia with Lewy bodies: a prospective clinical and neuropathological comparative study with Alzheimer's disease, *Am J Psychiatry* (1999) **156**:1039–45.

Ballard C, Piggott M, Johnson M et al, Delusions associated with elevated muscarinic binding in dementia with Lewy bodies, *Ann Neurol* (2000) **48**:868–76.

Ballard CG, O'Brien J, James I, Swann A, *Dementia: Management of Behavioural and Psychological Symptoms* (Oxford University Press: Oxford, 2001a).

Ballard CG, O'Brien JT, Swann AG et al, The natural history of psychosis and depression in dementia with Lewy bodies and Alzheimer's disease: persistence and new cases over 1 year of follow-up, *J Clin Psychiatry* (2001b) **62**:46–9.

Ballinger BR, Reid AH, Heather BB, Cluster analysis of symptoms in elderly demented patients, *Br J Psychiatry* (1982) **140**:257–62.

Binetti G, Padovani A, Magni E et al, Delusions and dementia: clinical CT correlates, *Acta Neurol Scand* (1995) **91**:271–275.

Birks JS, Harvey R, Donepezil for dementia due to Alzheimer's disease. Cochrane Dementia and Cognitive Improvement Group, *Cochrane Database of Systematic Reviews* (2004).

Brodaty H, Ames D, Snowdon J et al, A randomized placebo-controlled trial of risperidone for the treatment of aggression, agitation, and psychosis of dementia, *J Clin Psychiatry* (2003) **64**:134–43.

Burns A, Jacoby R, Levy R, Psychiatric phenomena in Alzheimer's Disease I-IV, *Br J Psychiatry* (1990) **157**:72–96.

Caligiuri MP, Peavy G, Salmon DP et al, Neuromotor abnormalities and risk for psychosis in Alzheimer's disease, *Neurology* (2003) **61**:954–8.

Chandler JD, Chandler JE, The prevalence of neuropsychiatric disorders in a nursing home population, *J Geriatr Psychiatry Neurol* (1988) **1**:71–6.

Chapman FM, Dickinson J, McKeith I, Ballard C, Association among visual hallucinations, visual acuity, and specific eye pathologies in Alzheimer's disease: treatment implications, *Am J Psychiatry* (1999) **156**:1983–5.

Chui HC, Lyness SA, Sobel E, Schneider LS, Extrapyramidal signs and psychiatric symptoms predict faster cognitive decline in Alzheimer's Disease, *Arch Neurol* (1994) **51**:676–81.

Cohen CI, Hyland K, Magai C, Inter-racial and intra-racial differences in neuropsychiatric symptoms, sociodemography and treatment among nursing home patients with dementia, *Gerontologist* (1998) **38**:355–61.

Cohen-Mansfield J, Nonpharmacologic interventions for psychotic symptoms in dementia, *J Geriatr Psychiatry Neurol* (2003) **16**:219–24.

Committee on Safety of Medicines, *Atypical Antipsychotic Drugs and Stroke*, 9 March 2004. [Available at: http://www.mca.gov.uk/aboutagency/regframework/csm/csmhome.htm]

Cooper JK, Mungas D, Weiler PG, Relation of cognitive status and abnormal behaviors in Alzheimer's disease, *J Am Geriatr Soc* (1990) **38**:867–70.

Cummings JL, Miller B, Hill MA, Neshkes R, Neuropsychiatric aspects of multi-infarct dementia and dementia of the Alzheimer type, *Arch Neurol* (1987) **44**:389–93.

Cummings JL, Mega M, Gray K et al, The Neuropsychiatric Inventory: comprehensive assessment of psychopathology in dementia, *Neurology* (1994) **44**:2308–14.

Deutsch LH, Bylsma FW, Rovner BW et al, Psychosis and physical aggression in probable alzheimers-disease, *Am J Psychiatry* (1991) **148**:1159–63.

Devanand DP, Miller L, Richards M et al, The Columbia University Scale for psychopathology in Alzheimer's disease, *Arch Neurol* (1992) **49**:371–6.

Drevets WC, Rubin EH, Psychotic symptoms and the longitudinal course of senile dementia of the Alzheimer type, *Biol Psychiatry* (1989) **25**:39–48.

Farber NB, Rubin EH, Newcomer JW et al, Increased neocortical neurofibrillary tangle density in subjects with Alzheimer disease and psychosis, *Arch Gen Psychiatry* (2000) **57**:1165–73.

Flynn GG, Cummings JL, Gorbein J, Delusions in dementia syndromes: investigation of behavioural and neuropsychological correlates, *J Neuropsychiatry Clin Neurosci* (1991) **3**:364–70.

Förstl H, Besthorn C, Geiger-Kabisch C et al, Psychotic features and the course of Alzheimer's disease: relationship to cognitive electroencephalographic and computerised tomography, *Acta Psychiatrica Scand* (1993) **87**:395–9.

Förstl H, Burns A, Levy R, Cairns N, Neuropathological correlates of psychotic phenomena in confirmed Alzheimer's disease, *Br J Psychiatry* (1994) **165**:53–9.

Gilley DW, Whalen ME, Wilson RS, Bennett DA, Hallucinations and associated factors in Alzheimer's disease, *J Neuropsychiatry* (1991) **3**:371–6.

Gilley DW, Wilson RS, Beckett LA, Evan DA, Psychotic symptoms and physically aggressive behavior in Alzheimer's disease, *J Am Geriatr Soc* (1997) **45**:1074–9.

Haupt M, Romero B, Kurz A, Psychotic symptoms in Alzheimer's disease: results from a two year longitudinal study, *Int J Geriatr Psychiatry* (1996) **11**:965–72.

Hirono N, Mori E, Yasuda M et al, Factors associated with psychotic symptoms in Alzheimer's disease, *J Neurol Neurosurg Psychiatry* (1998) **64**:648–52.

Holmes C, Smith H, Ganderton R et al, Psychosis and aggression in Alzheimer's disease: the effect of dopamine receptor gene variation, *J Neurol Neurosurg Psychiatry* (2001) **71**:777–9.

Holroyd S, Sheldon-Keller A, A study of visual hallucinations in Alzheimer's disease, *Am J Geriatr Psychiatry* (1995) **3**:198–205.

Hope T, Keene J, Fairburn C et al, Behavioural changes in dementia 2: are there behavioural syndromes?, *Int J Geriatr Psychiatry* (1997) **12**:1074–8.

Jeste DV, Wragg RE, Salmon DP et al, Cognitive deficits of patients with Alzheimer's disease with and without delusions, *Am J Psychiatry* (1992) **149**:184–9.

Jost BC, Grossberg GT, The evolution of psychiatric symptoms in Alzheimer's disease: a natural history study, *J Am Geriatr Soc* (1996) **44**:1078–81.

Katz IR, Jeste DV, Mintzer JE et al, Comparison of risperidone and placebo for psychosis and behavioral disturbances associated with dementia: a randomized, double-blind trial. Risperidone Study Group, *J Clin Psychiatry* (1999) **60**:107–15.

Lai MK, Lai OF, Keene J et al, Psychosis of Alzheimer's disease is associated with elevated muscarinic M2 binding in the cortex, *Neurology* (2001) **57**:805–11.

Lopez OL, Becker JT, Brenner RP et al, Alzheimers-disease with delusions and hallucinations – neuropsychological and electroencephalographic correlates, *Neurology* (1991) **41**:906–12.

Lopez OL, Gonzalez MP, Becker JT et al, Symptoms of depression and psychosis in Alzheimer's disease and frontotemporal dementia – exploration of underlying mechanisms, *Neuropsychiatry Neuropsychol Behav Neurol* (1996) **9**:154–61

Lyketsos CG, Steinberg M, Tschanz JT et al, Mental and behavioural disturbances in dementia: findings from the Cache County Study on Memory and Aging, *Am J Psychiatry* (2000) **157**:708–14.

McKeith IG, Fairbairn A, Perry R et al, Neuroleptic sensitivity in patients with senile dementia of Lewy body type, *BMJ* (1992). **305**:673–8.

McKeith I, Del Ser T, Spano P et al, Efficacy of rivastigmine in dementia with Lewy bodies: a randomised, double-blind, placebo-controlled international study, *Lancet* (2000) **356**:2031–6.

McShane R, Gedling K, Reading M et al, Prospective study of relations between cortical Lewy bodies, poor eyesight, and hallucinations in Alzheimer's Disease, *J Neurol Neurosurg Psychiatry* (1995) **59**:185–8.

McShane R, Keene J, Gedling K, Hope T, Hallucinations, cortical Lewy body pathology, cognitive function and neuroleptic use in dementia. In: Perry RH, McKeith IG, Perry EK, eds, *Dementia with Lewy Bodies* (Cambridge University Press: Cambridge, 1996).

Margallo-Lana M, Swann A, O'Brien J et al, (2001) Prevalence and pharmacological management of behavioural and psychological symptoms amongst dementia sufferers living in care environments, *Int J Geriatr Psychiatry* (2001) **16**:39–44.

Mega MS, Cummings JL, Fiorello T, Gornbein J, The spectrum of behavioral changes in Alzheimer's disease, *Neurology* (1996) **46**:130–5.

Migliorelli R, Petracca G, Teson A et al, Neuropsychiatric and neuropsychological correlates of delusions in Alzheimer's disease, *Psychol Med* (1995) **25**:505–13.

Mirza NR, Peters D, Sparks RG, Xanomeline and the antipsychotic potential of muscarinic receptor subtype selective agonists, *CNS Drug Rev* (2003) **9**:159–86.

Morriss RK, Rovner BW, Folstein MF, German PS, Delusions in newly admitted residents of nursing homes, *Am J Psychiatry* (1990) **147**:299–302.

Mortimer JA, Ebbitt B, Jun SP, Finch MD, Predictors of cognitive and functional progression in patients with probable Alzheimer's disease, *Neurology* (1992) **42**:1689–96.

Nacmias B, Tedde A, Forleo P et al, Association between 5-HT(2A) receptor polymorphism and psychotic symptoms in Alzheimer's disease, *Biol Psychiatry* (2001) **50**:472–5.

Olin J, Schneider L, Galantamine for dementia due to Alzheimer's disease. Cochrane Dementia and Cognitive Improvement Group, *Cochrane Database of Systematic Reviews* (2004).

Patterson MB, Schnell AH, Martin RJ et al, Assessment of behavioral and affective symptoms in Alzheimer's disease, *J Geriatr Psychiatry Neurol* (1990) **3**:21–30.

Paulsen J, Salmon D, Thal L et al, Incidence of and risk factors for hallucinations and delusions in patients with probable AD, *Neurology* (2000) **54**:1965–71.

Perry EK, Marshall E, Thompson P et al, Monoaminergic activities in Lewy body dementia: relation to hallucinations and extrapyramidal features, *J Neural Transm Park Dis Dement Sect* (1993) **6**:167–77.

Reisberg G, Borenstein J, Salob S et al, Behavioral symptoms in Alzheimer's disease: phenomenology and treatment, *J Clin Psychiatry* (1987) **47**:9–15.

Rockwell E, Jackson E, Vilke G, Jeste DV, A study of delusions in a large cohort of Alzheimer's disease patients, *Am J Psychiatry* (1994) **2**:157–64.

Rosen J, Zubenko GS, Emergence of psychosis and depression in the longitudinal evaluation of Alzheimer's disease, *Biol Psychiatry* (1991) **29**:2224–32.

Rovner BW, Kajonck S, Filipp L et al, The prevalence of mental illness in a community nursing home, *Am J Psychiatry* (1986) **143**:1446–9.

Rubin EH, Drevets WC, Burke WJ, The nature of psychotic symptoms in senile dementia of the Alzheimer type, *J Geriatr Psychiatry Neurol* (1988) **1**:16–20.

Schneider LS, Pollock VE, Lyness SA, A meta-analysis of controlled trials of neuroleptic treatment in dementia, *J Am Geriatr Soc* (1990) **38**:553–63.

Skoog I, The prevalence of psychotic, depressive, and anxiety syndromes in demented and non-demented 85 year olds, *Int J Geriatr Psychiatry* (1993) **8**:247–53.

Steele C, Rovner B, Chase GA, Folstein M, Psychiatric symptoms and nursing home placement of patients with Alzheimer's disease, *Am J Psychiatry* (1990) **147**:1049–51.

Street JS, Clark WS, Gannon KS et al, Olanzapine treatment of psychotic and behavioural symptoms in patients with Alzheimer disease in nursing care facilities: a double-blind, randomized, placebo-controlled trial. The HGEU Study Group, *Arch Gen Psychiatry* (2000) **57**:968–76.

Sultzer DL, Levin HS, Mahler ME et al, A comparison of psychiatric symptoms in vascular dementia and Alzheimer's disease, *Am J Psychiatry* (1993) **150**:1806–12.

Sweet RA, Hamilton RL, Lopez OL et al, Psychotic symptoms in Alzheimer's disease are not associated with more severe neuropathologic features, *Int Psychogeriatrics* (2000) **12**:547–58.

Tariot PN, CERAD behaviour rating scale for dementia, *Int Psychogeriatrics* (1996) **8** (Suppl 3):317–20; discussion 351–4.

Zubenko GS, Moossy J, Marinez AJ et al, Neuropathological and neurochemical correlates of psychosis in primary dementia, *Arch Neurol* (1991) **48**:619–24.

chapter 15

Psychotic symptoms and stress

Richard Bonwick

Introduction

Life expectancy and the total number of elderly people are steadily increasing in all developed countries. Psychiatric disorders in the elderly are recognized as a major contributor to mortality and morbidity. Psychotic symptoms, part of many common psychiatric disorders, are among the most distressing and disabling psychiatric symptoms encountered in any age group, and the elderly are no exception. An improved understanding of stress and its relationship with psychotic symptoms can only aid our attempts to optimize treatment, reduce disability, and alleviate suffering in many elderly patients. Post-traumatic stress disorder (PTSD), which frequently involves psychotic and psychotic-like symptoms, perhaps best exemplifies the intimate relationship between stress and psychiatric illness and warrants special attention in trying to better understand this topic.

What is stress?

The term stress, although widely used, can be confusing. Stress is most commonly defined as the nonspecific reaction an individual experiences in response to a perceived external threat. This response has physical, cognitive, and emotional components. Using this definition it is synonymous with stress reaction. Confusion arises as stress is also frequently used to describe the external threat. For clarity the external threat causing a stress reaction is better termed a stressor. To avoid perpetuating this confusion I will adhere to the terms stress reaction and stressor for the remainder of this chapter.

Stressors and mental illness in the elderly

In an elderly population the commonest, and most widely recognized, severe stressors would be the so-called loss events. These include significant events such as the loss of a partner, spouse or close friend through death; loss of physical integrity through illness; loss of independence or function through disability; and loss of meaningful activity through retirement.

Contemporary theory strongly associates these loss events in the elderly with the onset of neurotic disorders, such as depression (Murphy, 1982). However, stressors can trigger, or precipitate, a wide variety of psychological stress reactions in the elderly, possibly depending on the genetic vulnerability of the individual, and neurobiological factors (such as the presence of degenerative brain disease).

The recognition of the central role of a stressor in any type of mental illness has resulted in the inclusion of axis IV in the widely used multi-axial diagnostic system detailed most recently in the fourth edition of the Diagnostic and Statistical Manual of Mental Disorders (DSM-IV) (American Psychiatric Association, 1994). Axis IV allows a listing of stressors, termed psychosocial and environmental problems relevant to the primary (or axis I) diagnosis.

Psychiatric disorders in old age are no exception. Arguably all psychiatric disorders of old age, which typically include psychotic symptoms, can be understood to have an etiological association with a severe stressor. For example, an elderly patient with long-standing schizophrenic illness may respond to any minor perturbation in their environment, perceiving this as a significant stressor, by relapsing into an acute psychotic state. A patient may develop a psychotic depression after experiencing a severe personal stressor. Other examples may demonstrate a less direct, albeit equally significant, etiological association – an elderly patient with alcohol dependence may significantly increase or decrease alcohol consumption in response to a stressor, and precipitate an alcoholic hallucinosis or even a delirium tremens. A patient with dementia may develop psychotic symptoms seemingly in response to a stressful environmental change.

PTSD in the elderly

The psychiatric diagnosis most closely associated with a stressor is PTSD. It is unique within current diagnostic systems, being the only psychiatric condition including a specific stressor as part of its definition.

PTSD can occur in any age group, and is frequently a chronic and disabling anxiety disorder. The syndrome of PTSD consists of clusters of re-experiencing, avoidance/numbing, and arousal symptoms, etiologically related to a certain type of stressor, termed the traumatic event. The most widely accepted description of the necessary stressor occurs in DSM-IV, where it is defined as 'the person experienced, witnessed, or was confronted with an event or events that involved actual or threatened death or serious injury, or a threat to the physical integrity of self or others: and the person's response involved fear, helplessness or horror' (American Psychiatric Association, 1994).

The core symptoms of PTSD include re-experiencing the traumatic event via nightmares, intrusive daytime thoughts, or flashbacks, and even re-enacting the trauma in a real or symbolic manner. There is heightened arousal with generalized anxiety, irritability, insomnia, an exaggerated startle response, hyper-vigilance, and impaired concentration. Exposure to reminders of the trauma results in physiological reactivity and psychological distress. In response the sufferer actively avoids any potential reminders of the initial trauma, and may manifest an emotional numbness, a sense of foreshortened future and psychogenic amnesia of the initial trauma. In addition to these core symptoms a number of other symptoms are often encountered. These include dissociative episodes, survivor guilt (guilt at surviving a trauma when others did not), paranoid thinking, and rage attacks.

Psychotic symptoms and PTSD

Many patients with PTSD experience frank psychotic symptoms (delusions and hallucinations) with impaired reality testing and severely impaired ego function. In addition, phenomenologically many of the typical symptoms of PTSD have a psychotic quality.

Flashbacks are considered as intense forms of visual imagery, but frequently have a hallucinatory quality. During these the patient experiences visual images, related to their trauma, in brief snatches or greater complexity. Attached to this is the sense of being 'back there', and out of touch with current reality. Patients may re-enact the trauma, and behavior consistent with visual, auditory, and other hallucinations can be observed. Many sufferers, even during clear consciousness, will describe how they can still vividly smell, hear, and even see the stimuli attached to the traumatic event.

Cognitions surrounding survivor guilt can reach delusional intensity. Various cognitive distortions with a persecutory and paranoid theme may be so intense as to have a psychotic quality. This can be most apparent when the patient is confronted by a stressor that reminds them of their initial trauma in a real or symbolic way. They may even act on these paranoid beliefs when misinterpreting those around them as a tormentor or persecutor from their past. The severity and illogicality of rage attacks, an extreme manifestation of irritability, in response to even minor and trivial stimuli, suggests questionable reality testing.

The literature concerning psychotic symptoms in elderly PTSD sufferers is scant, but studies in younger adult populations identify the presence of psychotic symptoms in PTSD. One study found that up to 40% of patients with PTSD (following military combat trauma many decades earlier) had persisting psychotic symptoms, with auditory hallucinations being most common (David et al, 1999).

Acute PTSD in the elderly

Despite the increasing independence and longevity of the elderly in all developed countries, and a strongly held perception in the general community that the elderly are increasingly victims of crime, the issue of acute stress reactions to trauma, including PTSD, in elderly populations has been little studied. No studies allow even an estimate of prevalence figures within the community (Fields, 1996), but it is considered (perhaps incorrectly) a rare condition. Although acute reactions to traumatic events have enjoyed a burgeoning literature in recent years there has been limited focus on the elderly (Hyman, 1997). The few studies that have included the elderly suggest that as a group they experience similar phenomena to younger populations, with possibly an increased frequency of arousal symptoms, co-morbid depression, and sleep disturbance (Livingston et al, 1992). There is some evidence that increased age at the time of the trauma may in fact offer psychological protection (Weintraub and Ruskin, 1999). To date there has been no research published on the presence (or absence) of psychotic phenomena in acute PTSD in the elderly.

Chronic PTSD in the elderly

More commonly encountered in clinical practice with the elderly is chronic PTSD, often dating from traumatic events up to 70 years ago. This is particularly true for the current generation of elderly in the developed world, most of whom were involved directly or indirectly with World War II, which ended nearly 60 years ago. Best estimates suggest that 15% or more of elderly combat veterans, and an unknown number of civilians, continue to suffer with PTSD related to war-time trauma (Bonwick and Morris, 1996).

Chronic PTSD present for over five decades has a complex lifetime history. Core symptoms fluctuate in intensity and frequency, with arousal and re-experiencing symptoms being particularly persistent (Bonwick, 2002). In addition, chronic PTSD is frequently complicated by the sequential development of co-morbid psychiatric diagnoses through the life course (Davidson et al, 1990). The commonest of these are major depression, and alcohol abuse or dependence. Up to two-thirds of elderly chronic PTSD sufferers may have a lifetime diagnosis of major depression (Collier, 1999). Dysthymia, panic disorder, and other anxiety disorders are also common.

Research into the symptom profile of elderly people suffering chronic PTSD is exceedingly limited. In my clinical experience with large numbers of elderly Australian World War II veterans, whose PTSD stems from military service in their twenties, presentation with prominent psychotic symptoms is now uncommon. In particular dissociative symptoms and flashbacks, common in acute PTSD, tend to have persisted into middle-age, but have then burnt out. However, talking with these now elderly war veterans they describe psychotic symptoms in the years immediately following the war. The severity of these, and associated agitation, resulted in the use of heavy sedation, and seclusion in what they describe as 'padded cells'.

Occasionally elderly patients with PTSD still present with psychotic symptoms, but these are of a different nature. Even in recent years I have seen cases of elderly World War II veterans, with clear-cut lifelong PTSD and no previous history of an affective disorder, who in response to a new (and psychologically significant) stressor, have become manic, with psychotic symptoms.

The more common co-morbidities of chronic PTSD – major depression and alcohol abuse/dependence – may include psychotic symptoms, such as alcoholic hallucinosis. In my experience the quality of the depressive or alcohol-related psychotic symptoms is not influenced by the presence of an underlying chronic PTSD. These conditions, and their association with psychosis, are discussed elsewhere in this book.

These elderly patients with chronic PTSD may also additionally develop the typical psychiatric diagnoses of old age, including dementia and other neurodegenerative disorders. The presentation of dementia frequently includes psychotic symptoms. Although not widely studied, there is no evidence to suggest that the presence of chronic PTSD influences the onset of a dementing illness. However, the content of any psychotic symptoms may be determined by past traumas and chronic PTSD. For example, an elderly war veteran with chronic PTSD and dementia may have visual hallucinations of enemy soldiers or past persecutors.

Antipsychotic medication and treatment of PTSD

Although the use of antidepressant medication is the commonest treatment for PTSD, there is a time-honored practice of using antipsychotic medication (both oral and intramuscular). This dates back to the introduction of chlorpromazine. In particular antipsychotics have been, and continue to be, commonly used during the acute phases of the illness, and during exacerbations of symptoms which occur throughout the lifetime course of chronic PTSD.

Current practice would be to use atypical agents, because of a preferred side effect profile over more traditional antipsychotics. These medications are efficacious in alleviating frank psychotic symptoms, but also have an effect on other PTSD symptoms. It may simply be the sedative effect of this class of medications, but clinically the effect is often far more positive than when using other sedative agents, such as benzodiazepines.

A small number of placebo-controlled trials of atypical antipsychotic agents support their efficacy in PTSD (Stein et al, 2002). Within my unit there is a current research project examining the effects of the atypical antipsychotic, quetiapine, in PTSD (Hopwood, 2004, personal communication) but no results are available as yet. To date antipsychotic medication usage in the elderly with PTSD has received little research attention.

Post-psychosis PTSD

There is a growing literature in the adult populations that the traumatic experience of a psychotic episode and its associated treatment (including involuntary hospitalization) is a major stressor and may be followed by a form of PTSD (McGorry et al, 1991). This issue undoubtedly remains controversial, but assuming that the observation possesses some validity it raises interesting questions for a similar elderly patient group. First, does it also exist in this elderly population? Second, does the same phenomenon occur after an episode of psychotic depression, or dementia complicated by psychotic symptoms? Third, what role does cognitive integrity play in the development of post-psychosis PTSD – does cognitive impairment or dementia predispose in some way?

Conclusion

The association between stressors and psychotic symptoms in the elderly is important, with increasing clinical relevance in our aging developed societies. In particular PTSD, with its assumed etiological relationship with a traumatic stressor event, and its array of psychotic and psychotic-like symptoms, may offer many insights to this association. However, any possible understanding from studying this disease is hampered by a lack of meaningful research. In fact, there is currently a dearth of research concerning the whole topic of this chapter – psychotic symptoms and stress in the elderly. The subject, like many in old age psychiatry, awaits further exploration, and offers a rich, untapped vein for exploration by future researchers.

References

American Psychiatric Association, *Diagnostic and Statistical Manual of Mental Disorders*, 4th edn (DSM-IV) (American Psychiatric Association: Washington, DC, 1994).

Bonwick R, The Australian experience: post-traumatic stress disorder in the elderly, *IPA Bull* (2002) **19**:9–10.

Bonwick R, Morris P, Post-traumatic stress disorder in elderly war veterans, *Int J Geriatr Psychiatr* (1996) **11**:1071–6.

Collier P, Outcome study of an outpatient post-traumatic stress disorder group program for elderly war veterans. University of Melbourne Master of Medicine thesis (1999).

David D, Kucher G, Jackson E, Mellman T, Psychotic symptoms in combat-related posttraumatic stress disorder, *J Clin Psychiatry* (1999) **60**:29–32.

Davidson J, Kudler H, Saunders W, Smith R, Symptom and comorbidity patterns in World War II and Vietnam veterans with posttraumatic stress disorder, *Compr Psychiatry* (1990) **31**:162–70.

Fields R, Severe stress and the elderly: are older adults at increased risk of posttraumatic stress disorder. In: Ruskin P, Talbot J, eds, *Aging and Posttraumatic Stress Disorder* (American Psychiatric Association: Washington, DC, 1996) 79–100.

Hyman I, Post-traumatic stress disorder in the elderly. In: Black D, Newman M, Harris-Hendriks J, Mezey G, eds, *Psychological Trauma, a Developmental Approach* (Gaskell: London, 1997) 199–204.

Livingston H, Livingston M, Brooks D, McKinlay W, Elderly survivors of the Lockerbie air disaster, *Int J Geriatr Psychiatry* (1992) **7**:725–9.

McGorry P, Chanen A, McCarthy E et al, Posttraumatic stress disorder following recent-onset psychosis: an unrecognized postpsychotic syndrome, *J Nerv Ment Dis* (1991) **179**:640.

Murphy E, Social origins of depression in old age, *Br J Psychiatry* (1982) **141**:135–42.

Stein M, Kline N, Matloff J, Adjunctive olanzapine for SSRI-resistant combat-related PTSD, *Am J Psychiatry* (2002) **159**:1777–9.

Weintraub D, Ruskin P, Posttraumatic stress disorder in the elderly: a review, *Harv Rev Psychiatry* (1999) **7**:144–52.

chapter 16

Psychotic disorders with alcohol and substance abuse in the elderly

Greg Whelan

Clinical presentation

Mary Forthwright* – a 70-year-old widowed female who lived independently was discovered in a confused state by a neighbor who was alerted that all was not well by the presence of uncollected newspapers. Mary was confused, disorientated, dishevelled, agitated, and muttering that she was having trouble getting the cow into the cowshed. The neighbor, who could not see the cow, thought she was demented and called her family who took her to hospital. Although the family were aware that their mother had been drinking heavily for the last 10 years following the death of her farmer husband and Mrs Forthright's relocation to the city, they did not link it to her presentation and were too embarrassed to tell the Emergency Room staff.

Mary's hospital doctors were alerted to the diagnosis of alcohol withdrawal two days after admission when the social worker reported that her home visit revealed the presence of many empty gin bottles in the house.

Missing the diagnosis can be harmful

When presented with an elderly patient who is suffering a psychotic episode, in the absence of a positive history of substance abuse dependence, many clinicians will miss the diagnosis and fail to perform the appropriate investigations to confirm it.

* Pseudonym to protect patient identity.

The risk of iatrogenic addiction is particularly high for the elderly who smoke, drink or suffer from depression (Sanjuan and Langenbucher, 1999). The use of benzodiazepines can lead to accidental injuries, falls, and confusional states. Cognitive impairment resulting from the use of drugs and alcohol is particularly a problem for the elderly depressed since the clinical picture is often mistaken for irreversible dementia and inappropriate treatment is undertaken. Alcohol and benzodiazepine withdrawal is another particularly dangerous process for the elderly person, who may develop episodes of delirium and possibly withdrawal seizures. These withdrawal signs in the elderly may be attributed to infection or hypoxia and may result in under-treatment or inappropriate treatment.

In addition to psychotic symptoms directly due to substance abuse, the clinician needs to keep in mind that the patient may have co-morbid disorders, or mental health and substance abuse problems. A psychotic episode in an elderly individual who has an established diagnosis of dementia, depression or schizophrenia may be interpreted as a complication of one of these disorders rather than as substance-related.

The setting for substance abuse disorders in the elderly includes a continuation of a long-standing abuse/dependence problem or the development of such a problem in one whose life circumstances change – e.g. due to poor physical health, bereavement, depression, social isolation, and dementia. These situations in an elderly population can lead to increased use of alcohol and prescription and over-the-counter medication (Sanjuan and Langenbucher, 1999).

Failure to recognize that an acute psychotic episode in an elderly person is due to a substance use disorder may result in harm to that person. Untreated alcohol withdrawal can be complicated by seizures and dehydration. On the other hand, unnecessary exposure to neuroleptic treatment over a prolonged period of time may result in adverse reactions in a sensitive individual.

Which drugs are likely to cause psychosis in the elderly?

Alcohol

Older adults often experience alcohol-related consequences at lower levels of intake than younger adults (Chermack et al, 1996; Sanjuan and Langenbucher, 1999; Barry et al, 2001). Alcohol use disorders tend to be less prevalent in the elderly than those under 65 years (Sanjuan and Langenbucher, 1999; Lynsky et al, 2003). However, cognitive impairment may influence the accuracy of a history taken from an older adult. In addition, because of the stigma attached to problematic drinking, both the individual and the family may underestimate the elderly person's consumption or information related to alcohol use particularly may be missed as family members and even professional caregivers may conspire in the elderly person's denial of a problem (Sanjuan and Langenbucher, 1999). Adams and associates (1992) found that 14% of elderly emergency department patients were current alcohol abusers but were detected as such by their doctors in only 21% of cases.

Elderly individuals with alcohol use disorders are more likely to have an associated benzodiazepine dependence and nutritional deficiencies, particularly of folate and thiamine, when food intake is reduced because calories are derived from alcohol (Rigler, 2000). The development of cirrhosis carries a poor prognosis in the elderly (Smith, 1995). Other health problems related to alcohol abuse include drug interactions (Sanjuan and Langenbucher, 1999), hypertension, and stroke.

Alcohol withdrawal
Alcohol withdrawal can usually be recognized in the elderly by the presence of tremulousness in the presence of anxiety and agitation commencing soon (within hours) after ceasing drinking. Psychotic episodes such as transitory hallucinations are often manifested by seeing 'visions' of animals (which may be terrifying) or dead relatives (which may be disturbing). Appropriate treatment will allow the patient to settle and prevent the progression of the withdrawal to severe delirium and convulsions.

Benzodiazepines
The elderly are very large consumers of benzodiazepines, usually for the treatment of insomnia which itself may result from loneliness, inactivity, anxiety, boredom, and depression (O'Connor et al, 2001). Even low level use can lead to falls and confusion in the elderly.

Benzodiazepine withdrawal
Benzodiazepine withdrawal produces a characteristic sedative withdrawal pattern which includes anxiety, tremor, insomnia, nausea, and vomiting. It may be complicated by seizures and delirium (Wesson et al, 1997).

The withdrawal delirium may include disorientation as regards time, place, and situation. Auditory and visual hallucinations can complicate the picture. The delirium generally follows a period of insomnia. Occasionally patients will develop a protracted withdrawal syndrome. In addition to anxiety and sleep disturbance, these individuals may have increased sensitivity to light and sound as well as psychotic symptoms which may include hallucinations involving disturbance of smell.

The elderly may suffer unrecognized withdrawal from low dose prolonged benzodiazepine use.

Illicit drug use/abuse

Data from surveys indicate that use of drugs such as cannabis, amphetamines, heroin, and hallucinogens is uncommon in the elderly (Lynsky et al, 2003). When it does occur it is commonly missed.

Co-morbidity

Intoxication or withdrawal states due to substances can cause symptoms of mood as well as psychotic disorders. Substances may be used to manage mood, anxiety or psychotic disorders. Depressive symptoms are exceedingly common in substance abuse disorders and may well be diagnosed as primary mood disorders (Rosenthal and Westreich, 1999).

It has been recognized that an increased vulnerability to drug abuse can manifest itself through self-medication of states related to mental disorders. For example, the negative symptoms of schizophrenia may predispose affected individuals to subsequent substance abuse, particularly the stimulants such as amphetamines.

Standardized assessment will often reveal greater levels of substance abuse disorder in a psychiatric population than is noted with routine clinical procedures (Ananth et al, 1989). In a study performed in an inpatient dual diagnoses unit, Ananth and colleagues showed that substance abuse/dependence in schizophrenia patients occurred in almost 11% (abusing or dependent upon three or more substances) by retrospective chart review, 16% by routine clinical methods, and some 90% using structured research interviews. There is no published information to inform us whether these levels also occur in the elderly with schizophrenia.

Differential diagnosis

An elderly individual with substance-induced psychotic disorder may present in a manner that is clinically indistinguishable from any other psychotic disorder. Most patients with organic mental disorder (e.g. space-occupying lesions, epilepsy, infection, metabolic disorders, vascular disorders), are likely to have deficits in intellectual and cognitive functioning as a prominent feature. Where present these may be helpful. However, psychotic symptoms can make these intellectual functions difficult to test.

Psychotic symptoms are more likely to occur in those who present with delirium (acute organic mental disorder) in which perceptual disturbances including hallucinations are common (less often delusions are a feature). The elderly person who is either intoxicated or withdrawing from alcohol or other drugs may have psychotic symptoms as an isolated phenomenon or these symptoms may co-exist with other organic mental disorders. Newly developed psychotic symptoms in the elderly require a thorough assessment.

The delirious patient will often have reduced clarity or awareness of the environment and reduced capacity to sustain attention. Some may be incoherent. It may be difficult to test memory or orientation. Symptoms may fluctuate over a short period and throughout the course of the day. When delusions are a prominent part of the presentation drugs such as amphetamines, cannabis or hallucinogens must be considered. This is far less likely to occur in the elderly but disorders such as temporal lobe epilepsy and nondominant cerebral lesions need consideration.

Assessment

A sensitively taken history from family or carers, particularly stressing the importance of obtaining an accurate alcohol or drug use history, is a critical part of making the diagnosis in a psychotic elderly individual.

Physical examination can be used to support a diagnosis of alcohol-related psychosis. Wernicke's encephalopathy – confusion, nystagmus, ophthalmoplegia and ataxia – would point to such a diagnosis and requires immediate and specific therapy with thiamine replacement. Evidence of liver disease or other organ damage is likely to indicate long-standing alcohol abuse/ dependence and can be helpful in this setting.

Simple laboratory tests such as full blood count, liver function tests, and a urinary drug screen can be helpful in supporting the diagnosis. It may, however, be critical to check for or to rule out other disorders – thyroid function tests, imaging of the brain, measurement of electrolytes, blood glucose (hypoglycemia), and renal function may be indicated by the clinical picture. In all patients, suicide risk should be assessed and appropriate measures taken to reduce the risk.

Treatment of alcohol and other substance use disorders in the elderly

Management of drug-related psychosis

Because intoxication or withdrawal can induce psychotic states or exacerbate pre-existing psychotic symptoms, acute psychosis is best handled symptomatically with safety being the primary concern. This usually means administering sedative medication such as diazepam for psychotic agitation (the treatment of choice in alcohol withdrawal) and deferring the use of antipsychotic medication until the clinical picture is clear.

In a presentation with a high probability of being drug-induced psychosis, benzodiazepines are the drug of choice. One needs to be aware that the metabolism of these drugs may be slow in the elderly and in those with significant liver disease. A dose adequate to control agitation (e.g. 40 mg or more diazepam daily) should be given prior to instituting antipsychotic medication.

Once a presumptive diagnosis of a psychotic disorder with persistent symptoms is made – whether related to substance use or not – treatment with an antipsychotic medication is warranted. In patients with severe mental disorders and substance abuse disorders compliance with medication is essential for stabilization.

Once the psychotic episode is under control consideration needs to be given to managing the underlying cause.

Relapse prevention in alcohol dependence

Even long-term alcohol abusers can be persuaded to stop drinking if the adverse effects are clearly explained to them. Mood disorders such as depression and anxiety must be tackled directly (O'Connor et al, 2001). Amelioration of loneliness and bereavement counselling may play an important role (O'Connor et al, 2001).

Many of the forms of therapy that are helpful for younger adults with alcohol problems are also of value in the elderly (Barry et al, 2001). Intrapersonal conflict such as depression, loneliness, loss, and social isolation are more likely to lead to relapse in the elderly than in younger people. Cognitive behavioral therapy appears to be just as effective for older adults as it is for those in younger age groups (Dupree et al, 1984; Barry et al, 2001). Tailoring groups to older adults may even be more beneficial than in younger people. Johnson (1989) reports that older adults preferred elderly-specific groups held at a relatively slow pace. Because they are well tolerated, medications such as naltrexone and acamprosate ought to be of some help. Of these drugs, naltrexone as an adjunct to therapy has been found to be well tolerated and to prevent relapse (Oslin et al, 1997). Disulfiram is usually avoided because of the high likelihood of vascular disorder in the elderly age group and the risk of precipitating stroke in this age group if an alcohol–disulfiram reaction occurs.

The management of benzodiazepine abuse

The elderly are very large consumers of benzodiazepines, usually for the treatment of insomnia which itself may result from loneliness, inactivity, anxiety, boredom, and depression. If sleep difficulties can be managed with sleep hygiene or without benzodiazepines many of the elderly would not suffer from secondary benzodiazepine abuse dependence issues. To manage benzodiazepine dependence in patients with established physical dependence, the usual therapeutic approach is to substitute a long-acting benzodiazepine (such as diazepam) and to gradually withdraw the substituted medication. Abrupt withdrawal of high dose benzodiazepines can be fatal if convulsions occur. The starting dose of diazepam to stabilize the patient will depend on patient tolerance. Most elderly patients (unless suffering concomitant alcohol dependence) will have 'low dose dependence' (Wesson et al, 1997) and can be stabilized on 15–20 mg diazepam prior to commencing gradual withdrawal over weeks or months. For those with very high tolerance, a dose of 60 mg daily will prevent withdrawal seizures and is a reasonable stabilization dose.

Alternatively, both carbamazepine (Schweizer et al, 1991) and valproate (Roy-Byrne et al, 1989) are effective in suppressing benzodiazepine withdrawal symptoms and do not carry risk of abuse.

Summary

Alcohol and benzodiazepine abuse/dependence in the elderly can be associated with psychotic symptoms, particularly in the context of drug intoxication or withdrawal. The diagnosis is often missed when there is a low incidence of suspicion or when the history of abuse is not elicited from carers or relatives. Diazepam is the medication of choice in suppressing psychotic agitation. A thorough assessment, attention to the management of predisposing factors, and relapse prevention approaches will often produce a sustained remission of the substance abuse disorder.

References

Adams WL, Mogruder-Habib K, Trued S, Broome HL, Alcohol abuse in elderly emergency department patients, *J Am Geriatr Soc* (1992) **40**:1236–40.

Ananth J, Vandeater S, Kamal M, Brodsky A, Missed diagnosis of substance abuse in psychiatric patients, *Hosp Community Psychiatry* (1989) **40**:297–9.

Barry KL, Oslin DW, Blow FC, *Alcohol Problems in Older Adults* (Springer Publishing: New York, 2001).

Chermack ST, Blow FC, Hill EM, The relationship between alcohol symptoms and consumption among older drinkers, *Alcohol Clin Exp Res* (1996) **20**:1153–8.

Dupree L, Broskowski H, Scholfeld L, The gerontology alcohol project: a behavioural program for elderly alcohol abusers, *Gerontologist* (1984) **24**:510–16.

Johnson L, How to diagnose and treat chemical dependency in the elderly, *J Gerontol Nurs* (1989) **15**:22–6.

Lynsky MT, Day C, Hall W, Alcohol and other drug use disorders among older aged people, *Drug Alcohol Rev* (2003) **22**:125–33.

O'Connor D, Ames D, Chiu E, The psychiatry of old age. In Bloch S, Singh BS, eds, *Foundations of Clinical Psychiatry,* 2nd edn (Melbourne University Publishing: Melbourne, 2001) 439–61.

Oslin D, Liberto J, O'Brien J, Naltrexone as an adjunctive treatment for older patients with alcohol dependence, *Am J Geriatr Psychiatry* (1997) **5**:324–32.

Rigler SK, Alcoholism in the elderly, *Am Fam Physician* (2000) **261**:1710–16.

Rosenthal RN, Westreich L, Treatment of persons with dual diagnoses of substance use disorder and other psychological problems. In: McCready BS, Epstein EE, eds, *Addictions: a Comprehensive Guide Book* (Oxford University Press: Oxford, 1999) 439–76.

Roy-Byrne PP, Ward NG, Donnelly P, Valproate in anxiety and withdrawal syndromes, *J Clin Psychiatry* (1989) **50**:44–8.

Sanjuan PM, Langenbucher JW, Age-limited population: youth, adolescents and older adults. In: McCrady BS, Epstein EE, eds, *Addictions: A Comprehensive Guidebook* (Oxford University Press: Oxford, 1999) 497–8.

Schweizer E, Rickels K, Case WG, Greenblatt DJ, Carbamazepine treatment in patients discontinuing long term benzodiazepine therapy: effects on withdrawal severity and outcome, *Arch Gen Psychiatry* (1991) **48**:448–52.

Smith JW, Medical manifestations of alcoholism in the elderly, *Int J Addictions* (1995) **30**:1749–98.

Wesson DR, Smith ED, Ling W, Seymour R, Sedative hypnotics & tricyclics. In: Lowinson JH, Ruiz P, Millman RB, Langrod JG, eds, *Substance Abuse: a Comprehensive Textbook,* 3rd edn (Williams & Wilkins: Baltimore, 1997) 223–30.

chapter 17

Psychosis in the elderly – co-morbidity and disability: focus on basal ganglia diseases

Edmond Chiu

Introduction

Neuropsychiatric symptoms are frequent in many medical conditions. The conceptual questions of co-morbidity or causal relationships are often raised and challenge clinicians and researchers to seek for but not always succeed in reaching clarification. Nevertheless the co-existence of psychotic symptoms with medical illnesses gives rise to excess disability in patients, and adds a degree of complexity to the management of these medical illnesses.

The early studies of Berrios and Brook (1984) and Cummings (1985) threw light on the relationship between psychotic symptoms of delusions and hallucinations and medical conditions, prescribed drugs and toxic agents.

Cummings (1985) documented some 70 conditions implicated in the production of delusions. Central nervous system (CNS) disorders, in particular of the basal ganglia, temporal limbic regions, lesions of the temporal lobes and subcortical regions have been implicated. While neoplastic and vascular lesions impacting on these areas are readily understood through the neuroanatomical correlations of these destructive lesions, the occurrence of psychotic symptoms in basal ganglia diseases such as Parkinson's disease, basal ganglia calcification, and Huntington's disease has added to the understanding of the evolution of psychotic symptoms co-occurring with these pathologies, contributes to current knowledge of the role of the basal ganglia in psychotic symptoms, and leads to the conceptualization of the spectrum 'Lewy bodies disorders' (Hishikawa et al, 2003).

A paper in the *British Journal of Psychiatry* by Albert West (1973) described a pair of 24-year-old identical twins suffering an unspecified basal ganglia disorder who were psychiatrically normal before, who simultaneously developed a schizophrenia-like psychosis. West suggested that psychological stress might have disturbed an already impaired neurophysiology, producing the psychosis. Francis (1979) presented case histories to illustrate an association between familial basal ganglia calcification and schizophreniform symptomatology and suggested that the slow development of calcification could result in the development of schizophreniform psychosis and extrapyramidal symptoms presenting in adulthood. A link between basal ganglia pathology and psychosis was further suggested by Bowman and Lewis (1980), who analysed 22 diseases that have common symptoms with schizophrenia. These diseases include carbon monoxide poisoning, delirium tremens, Parkinson's disease (PD), and Wernicke's encephalopathy. In an effort to discern possible common sites of neuropathology, they identified an unusual degree of involvement of the basal ganglia with such diseases.

Cummings (1983), reporting a case of idiopathic calcification of the basal ganglia, also supported Francis in the development of psychosis in early adulthood. Presentations later in life include dementia and a motor system disorder. He further suggested that subcortical structural pathology could produce schizophrenia-like symptoms that may precede the onset of intellectual deterioration and extrapyramidal motor disorder.

Cummings (1985), in his analysis of psychotic systems in medical conditions, made the connection between these symptoms in the pathology of limbic and basal ganglia areas which are predisposed to abnormal emotional experiences which when interpreted by the intact cortex lead to complex and well-structured delusions. The similarity to schizophrenia may be related to the disruption of ascending dopaminergic pathways by subcortical and limbic lesions in the CNS diseases.

In a prospective study of 102 consecutive patients diagnosed by strictly defined criteria for PD, Holroyd et al (2001) identified four with psychosis due solely to delirium. Of the remaining 98 patients, 30 had hallucinations or delusions; 26 had visual hallucinations; two had auditory hallucinations; one also had delusions and one had gustatory hallucinations. Visual hallucinations were significantly associated with worse visual acuity, lower cognitive score, higher depression score, and worse disease severity. However, history of psychiatric disorder, dose or duration of levodopa or other anti-parkinsonian medication treatment or duration of illness were not associated with hallucinations.

Barnes and David (2001), in the same issue of the same journal, reported that in their case-controlled study, hallucinations in PD were associated with greater age and duration and severity of illness, cognitive impairment, sleep disturbance, and depression. They described the complex visual images experienced by the hallucinators as resembling those highlighted in hallucinations of the visually impaired.

The editorial (Mindham, 2001) which commented on these papers contended that, since the central category of idiopathic PD is diminishing and the boundaries between neurodegenerative diseases are becoming less distinct, the diagnosis of the disease is becoming increasingly problematic. Hallucinations may be a nonspecific response to a range of circumstances in conditions that predispose to their occurrence. This being the case, the elderly with both PD and psychotic symptoms may possess a common, albeit sometimes distinct, biological (neurodegenerative) pathology finding a final common pathway in their clinical expression.

Psychotic symptoms in PD

Prevalence and risk factors

As diseases of the basal ganglia, in particular PD, are common in the elderly, an exploration of this medical condition and its relationship to psychotic symptoms and consequent excess disability will be the focus of this chapter.

In a sample of 43 patients with PD, Haeske-Dewick (1995) described 10 subjects (23%) who reported hallucinations. However, when interviewed, 16/36 (44%) subjects were identified to have been hallucinating. Age, disability stage, self-reported sensory loss, and cognitive decline were significantly greater in those experiencing hallucinations. Care burden was noted to be related to severity of depression. However, premorbid intelligence, daily levodopa intake, and the use of other anti-parkinsonian medication did not discriminate those with hallucinations from those who were not hallucinating.

Goetz and Stebbins (1995) studied 11 subjects (mean age = 75.6) with advanced PD who entered nursing homes over a period of five years. All were dead within two years after the study. Compared with 22 community-dwelling subjects who were alive at the end of the study, the presence of hallucinations, not motor or intellectual impairment, was related to both admission to nursing homes and mortality. This small study, despite its methodological defects, does point to a possible relationship between the presence of hallucinations and increased nursing home admissions and subsequent mortality.

Aarsland et al (1999a) in a population-based study of 235 patients with PD reported a frequency of hallucinations and delusions of 16%; especially common in the late phases of the illness. This group of patients also showed more dementia, depression, severe motor changes, and atypical clinical features. They suggested that such extensive and more severe clinical features are related to more advanced and widespread brain changes involving critical neurotransmitter systems underlying the emergence of psychotic symptoms in patients with PD.

A study of 216 consecutive patients (mean age = 69) fulfilling clinical criteria for PD was reported by Fenelon et al (2000). Hallucinations were identified as being present for the previous three months in 39.8% of the patients. These hallucinations could be classified into three categories:

1. 'Minor' forms consisting of a sensation of a presence of a person, or an animal, or illusions were present in 25.5% of patients.
2. Formed visual hallucinations were present in 22.2%. of patients.
3. Auditory hallucinations were present in 9.7% of patients.

Those with 'minor forms' had higher depression scores than nonhallucinators. Logistic regression analysis identified three factors that were independently predictive of formed visual hallucinations: severe cognitive disorders, daytime somnolence, and a long duration of PD. It was further noted that when 'minor' hallucinations were included, the total prevalence was much higher than previously reported.

For patients who had PD with dementia (PDD), Naimark et al (1996) found 36 of 101 PDD patients to have either hallucinations, delusions, or both. These individuals were also found to have more insomnia, confusion, agitation, personality changes, and self-care problems, and were reported by their carers to be more difficult to manage at home. Cognitively, they were more impaired than the nonpsychotic subjects. Psychotic symptoms in PDD were associated with more disability in major behavioral, cognitive, and functional domains.

The role of dopamine in psychotic symptoms in PD

Celesia and Barr (1970) reported that among 45 patients receiving oral levodopa therapy, 16/45 patients developed psychoses, acute anxiety, euphoria, and other neuropsychiatric phenomena, and of these 16 patients 14 also developed generalized dyskinesia. These psychotic symptoms emerged only after several weeks of maintenance therapy on a previously well-tolerated dose. This report suggested that catecholamine and other brain monoamines might be implicated.

Friedhoff and Alpert (1973) proposed the theory that an increase in dopaminergic activity or a decrease in cholinergic activity produces psychotic symptoms but relieves parkinsonian symptoms. Conversely, a decrease of dopaminergic activity or an increase of cholinergic activity relieves psychotic symptoms but produces more parkinsonian symptoms. This raises a significant clinical dilemma for physicians treating PD.

Subsequently, Cummings (1991) summarized information regarding behavior disturbances associated with PD treatment. He reported that a variety of neuropharmacologic agents, including anticholinergic drugs, amantadine, levodopa, selegiline, bromocriptine, and pergolide when administered in excessive doses or to susceptible individuals may produce alterations in mood, thought content, attention, personal security, or sexual behavior. Moreover, major behavioral disturbances observed during the course of PD treatment include hallucinations, delusions, mania, hypomania, euphoria, depression, anxiety, altered sexual behavior, and confusion. He considered these a consequence of the therapy when they appear for the first time soon after initiation of treatment or after an increase in drug dosage. The reduction of dosage or discontinuation of drugs will improve the behavior disorders.

A contrary view has been expressed by Cannas et al (2001), who studied a small sample of seven patients with early-onset PD who had developed psychiatric manifestations consisting of chronic delusional hallucinatory psychosis after a few years of anti-parkinsonian therapy. They suggested, after thorough cognitive, neurological, and neuroimaging explorations, that these patients with early-onset PD, normal or slight cognitive impairment, and normal computed tomography/magnetic resonance imaging brain scans had the expression of a co-existing psychotic illness, which prior to onset of the neurological disease had not been correctly diagnosed and which had been disclosed by dopaminergic therapy.

The problem of pharmacologically induced excess disability

The primary motor symptoms of PD and other basal ganglia disorders have a critical role in the disability suffered by elderly patients. Mobility disturbances, increased frequency of falls, and reduction in independence through the loss of activity of daily living functions, all contribute to an increased requirement for supportive care and even early institutionalization. When psychotic symptoms are added to this mix, the excess disability so engendered will lead both to further disability for the elderly patients, and distress and an increased care burden for their carers. This situation of 'triple whammy' demands from the physician more effective ways of reducing or removing the psychotic symptoms, thus relieving the symptom burden in the patient and reducing carer stress, without increasing the motor or cognitive disability.

Anti-parkinsonian therapy is frequently related to the development of psychoses (Friedman and Sienkiewicz, 1991), as a recognized adverse consequence of treatment of motor symptoms. While reduction of the dose of anti-parkinsonian therapy may reduce the psychotic symptoms, it usually leads to aggravation of the motor symptoms – a 'catch 22' situation of less than satisfactory outcome.

The first-generation antipsychotics, while efficacious in the treatment of psychotic symptoms, will aggravate the motor symptoms. This strategy is now generally considered unacceptable. Following the arrival of the second-generation antipsychotics, which do not have the same level of extrapyramidal side effects as the first-generation antipsychotics, many studies have reported on their usefulness in the treatment of psychotic symptoms in PD.

Reports on *Clozapine* indicate that a low dosage (i.e. compared with dosage for treatment-resistant schizophrenia) of 6.25 mg or 12.5 mg per day can be effective (Factor et al, 1994; Chacko et al, 1995; Meltzer et al, 1995; Rabey et al, 1995).

Ondansetron, a 5-HT3 receptor antagonist, has been reported to be useful in 16 advanced PD patients with psychosis of 6–60 months' duration (Zoldan et al, 1995) without aggravating basic PD symptoms or levodopa efficacy and was well tolerated with no major side effects.

Olanzapine has also been studied (Wolters et al, 1996; Aarsland et al, 1999b), showing efficacy in both demented and nondemented subjects without worsening of parkinsonism or cognition. However, in the study by Aarsland and colleagues (1999b) drowsiness was responsible for treatment discontinuation in 29% of subjects. Marsh et al (2001) reported an open-label six-week trial of olanzapine in PDD and psychosis. There was no improvement in psychotic symptoms, and functional disability declined significantly. They concluded that olanzapine appears to be poorly tolerated in patients with PD, psychotic symptoms, and dementia.

Workman et al (1997) reported the use of *risperidone* in nine patients, 66–78 years of age, with PDD. There was a reduction in agitation and psychotic symptoms, without worsening of extrapyramidal symptoms, further cognitive impairment, or a need to increase anti-dyskinetic medication.

Quetiapine, a dibenzothiazepine atypical antipsychotic with a close pharmacological resemblance to clozapine, may offer an effective alternative treatment in this group of patients without compromising motor function (Matheson and Lamb, 2000). A case report by Weiner et al (2000) described an 81-year-old man with a 14-year history of PD and levodopa-induced psychosis who did not respond to olanzapine, but responded to 100 mg per day of quetiapine with complete resolution of hallucinations and delusions, without increase of motor symptoms. With regard to antipsychotic-naïve patients, Targum and Abbott (2000) reported that 11 patients with PD and acute psychosis, who were receiving dopaminergic agents, responded to quetiapine. Visual hallucinations were effectively controlled in six patients, but delusions were less responsive. Four patients withdrew due to adverse events or co-morbid medical problems, and two were withdrawn due to lack of efficacy. Quetiapine did not aggravate motor symptoms.

As a cholinergic mechanism may be partially involved in the hallucinations and delusions encountered in basal ganglia diseases such as PD, *donepezil* has been studied for the treatment of psychotic symptoms in patients with PD. Bergman and Lerner (2002) and Fabbrini et al (2002) reported preliminary open-label use of donepezil in this group of patients. Bergman and Lerner's (2002) six patients with PDD complicated by psychosis were treated with up to 10 mg/day of donepezil. Five patients had clinical improvement of psychotic symptoms, and one had minimal improvement after six weeks of treatment. No side effects or deterioration in parkinsonian symptoms were reported. Fabbrini et al (2002) reported significant improvement of hallucinations and delusions in all eight subjects with PD. However, motor disability deteriorated in two of the eight subjects.

With advances in psychopharmacology and the availability of novel antipsychotics and cholinesterase inhibitors, the future for the treatment of psychotic symptoms in PD with or without dementia is looking optimistic. With a reduction of added disability from psychotic symptoms, together with multidisciplinary psychosocial support for PD patients and their carers, we can anticipate a much better quality of life for them.

References

Aarsland A, Larsen JP, Cummings JL, Laake K, Prevalence and clinical correlates in psychiatric symptoms in Parkinson's disorder: a community based study, *Arch Neurol* (1999a) **56**:595–601.

Aarsland D, Larsen JP, Lim NG, Tandberg E, Olanzapine for psychosis in patients with Parkinson's disease with and without dementia, *J Neuropsychiatry Clin Neurosci* (1999b) **11**:392–4.

Barnes J, David AS, Visual hallucinations in Parkinson's disease: a review and phenomenological survey, *J Neurol Neurosurg Psychiatry* (2001) **70**:727–33.

Bergman J, Lerner V, Successful use of donepezil for the treatment of psychotic symptoms in patients with Parkinson's disease, *Clin Neuropsychopharmacol* (2002) **25**:107–10.

Berrios GE, Brook P, Visual hallucinations and sensory delusions in the elderly, *Br J Psychiatry* (1984) **144**:662–4.

Bowman M, Lewis MS, Sites of subcortical damage in diseases which resemble schizophrenia, *Neuropsychologia* (1980) **18** (4–5):597–601.

Cannas A, Spissu A, Floris GL et al, Chronic delusional hallucinatory psychosis in early onset Parkinson's disease: drug-induced complication or sign of an idiopathic psychiatric illness, *Neurol Sci* (2001) **22**:53–4.

Celesia GG, Barr AN, Psychosis and other psychiatric manifestations of levodopa therapy, *Arch Neurol* (1970) **23**:193–200.

Chacko RC, Hurley RA, Harper RG et al, Clozapine for acute and maintenance treatment of psychosis in Parkinson's disease, *J Neuropsychiatry Clin Neurosci* (1995) **7**:471–5.

Cummings JL, Neuropsychiatric disturbances associated with idiopathic calcification of the basal ganglia, *Biol Psychiatry* (1983) **18**:591–601.

Cummings JL, Organic delusions: phenomenology, anatomical correlation, and review, *Br J Psychiatry* (1985) **146**:184–97.

Cummings JL, Behavioral complications of drug treatment of Parkinson's disease, *J Am Geriatr Soc* (1991) **39**:708–16.

Fabbrini G, Barbanti P, Aurilia C et al, Donepezil in the treatment of hallucinations and delusions in Parkinson's disease, *Neurol Sci* (2002) **23**:41–3.

Factor SA, Brown D, Molho EC, Podskalny GD, Clozapine: a 2-year open trial in Parkinson's disease patients with psychosis, *Neurology* (1994) **44**:544–6.

Fenelon G, Mahieux F, Huon R, Ziegler M, Hallucinations in Parkinson's disease: prevalence, phenomenology and risk factors, *Brain* (2000) **123**:733–45.

Francis AF, Familial basal ganglia calcification and schizophreniform psychosis, *Br J Psychiatry* (1979) **135**:360–2.

Friedhoff AJ, Alpert M, A dopaminergic cholinergic mechanism in production of psychotic symptoms, *Biol Psychiatry* (1973) **62**:165–9.

Friedman A, Sienkiewicz J, Psychotic complications of long-term levodopa treatment of Parkinson's disease, *Acta Neurol Scand* (1991) **84**:111–13.

Goetz CG, Stebbins GT, Mortality and hallucinations in nursing homes with advanced Parkinson's disease, *Neurology* (1995) **45**:669–71.

Haeske-Dewick HC, Hallucinations in Parkinson's disease: characteristics and associated clinical features, *Int J Geriatr Psychiatry* (1995) **10**:487–95.

Hishikawa N, Hashizume Y, Yoshida M, Sobue G, Clinical and neuropathological correlates of Lewy body's disease, *Acta Neuropathol* (2003) **105**:341–50.

Holroyd S, Currie L, Wooten GF, Prospective study of hallucinations and delusions in Parkinson's disease, *J Neurol Neurosurg Psychiatry* (2001) **70**:734–8.

Marsh L, Lyketos C, Reich SG, Olanzapine for the treatment of psychosis in patients with Parkinson's disease and dementia, *Psychosomatics* (2001) **42**:477–81.

Matheson AJ, Lamb HM, Quetiapine: a review of its clinical potential in the management of psychotic symptoms in Parkinson's disease, *CNS Drugs* (2000) **14**:157–72.

Meltzer HY, Kennedy J, Dai J et al, Plasma clozapine levels and the treatment of L-dopa-induced psychosis in Parkinson's disease: a high potency effect of clozapine, *Neuropsychopharmacology* (1995) **12**:39–45.

Mindham RH, Visual hallucinations in Parkinson's disease: their nature, frequency and origins, *J Neurol Neurosurg Psychiatry* (2001) **70**:719–20.

Naimark D, Jackson E, Rockwell E, Jeste DV, Psychotic symptoms in Parkinson's disease patients with dementia, *J Am Geriatr Soc* (1996) **44**:296–9.

Rabey JM, Treves TA, Neufeld MY et al, Low dose clozapine in the treatment of levodopa-induced mental disturbances in Parkinson's disease, *Neurology* (1995) **45**:432–4.

Targum SD, Abbott JL, Efficacy of quetiapine in Parkinson's patients with psychosis, *J Clin Psychopharmcol* (2000) **20**:54–60.

Weiner WJ, Minager A, Shulman LM, Quetiapine for L-dopa-induced psychosis in PD, *Neurology* (2000) **54**:1538.

West A, Concurrent schizophrenic-like psychosis in monozygotic twins suffering from CNS disorder, *Br J Psychiatry* (1973) **122**:675–7.

Wolters E Ch, Jansen ENH, Tuynman-Qua HG, Bergmans PLM, Olanzapine in the treatment of dopaminergic psychosis inpatients with Parkinson's disease, *Neurology* (1996) **47**:1085–7.

Workman RH Jr, Orengo CA, Bakey AA et al, The use of risperidone for psychosis and agitation in demented patients with Parkinson's disorder, *J Neuropsychiatry Clin Neurosci* (1997) **9**:594–7.

Zoldan J, Friedberg G, Livneh M, Melamed E, Psychosis in advanced Parkinson's disease: treatment with ondensetron, a 5HT3 receptor antagonist, *Neurology* (1995) **45**:1305–8.

chapter 18

Iatrogenic psychosis

James S. Olver and Trevor R. Norman

Introduction

The physician's Hippocratic responsibilities include beneficence and non-maleficence; however, when managing the complex physiology of the human being, redressing pathology in one system invariably results in pseudopathological change in another. There are few treatments in medicine that are free of side effects. This process has been termed iatrogenesis (Greek: from or caused by the physician). Nowhere is this more apparent than in the fragile metabolic balance seen in the elderly where homeostatic responses are blunted and there is less metabolic reserve. One common constellation of adverse events seen in conjunction with medication treatments involves the impairment of reality testing, usually reflected by the development of perceptual abnormalities and delusional thoughts – often loosely termed 'psychosis'. In this chapter, we will outline the nomenclature of the 'iatrogenic psychoses', review some common drug-related and nondrug-related psychoses and discuss important changes in the physiology and pharmacology of the elderly that may underpin the 'iatrogenic psychoses'.

Classification and epidemiology

The epidemiology of medication-related psychosis is markedly limited by methodological problems. Large variations in incidence and prevalence data are most probably related to poorly defined diagnostic criteria and variability in patient populations sampled. Modern established diagnostic manuals have essentially approached the classification of iatrogenic psychosis in similar ways. Patients with impaired reality orientation as shown by perceptual abnormalities are divided into two groups: those with disturbances of consciousness and attention are diagnosed with delirium (substance-induced delirium in DSM-IV [American Psychiatric Association, 1994]), while those without are determined to have another organic disturbance (substance-induced psychotic disorder in DSM-IV or organic hallucinosis or organic delusional disorder in ICD-10 [WHO, 1992]). It is, however, unlikely that subtle neurocognitive disturbances are absent in the nondelirium diagnostic categories and that a spectrum of cognitive disturbances exists between the two groups. The epidemiologic literature is dominated by single or small group case studies in which clinical descriptions are given, thus avoiding taxonomic arguments, and larger studies of medically ill patients where the diagnosis of delirium is sought according to established clinical criteria. Unless otherwise stated, no distinction will be made between delirious and nondelirious psychotic reactions in this chapter.

With these limitations in mind, studies using contemporary criteria for diagnosing delirium have shown high prevalence rates in the elderly. O'Keefe and Lavan (1997) reported that 18% of patients showed evidence of delirium on admission to an acute geriatric ward and a further 24% developed delirium during the admission. Most studies suggest that the rate is between 14% and 21% (Bucht et al, 1999). The etiology of delirium is frequently multifactorial and sometimes unknown and so few studies have attempted to separate out the number of subjects with medication-related delirium. The common causes of delirium are shown in Box 18.1. In a prospective study of elderly hospitalized patients, Francis et al (1990) reported that 50 of 229 (22%) developed a delirium attributable to medication, while Moore and O'Keefe (1999) suggested that the rate was as high as 30%, making drugs the third most common cause of delirium in elderly inpatients after electrolyte disturbance and infections. A wide variety of drugs have been implicated and, since the literature is primarily reliant on case reports, there is a bias to increased reports of older drugs. Drugs at high and medium risk of inducing delirium are listed in Box 18.2.

Box 18.1 Common causes of delirium

Metabolic/electrolyte disturbances
Infections – especially systemic, e.g. chest, urine
Drug intoxications
Drug withdrawals
Focal/diffuse neurological lesions
Pain
Constipation/urinary retention
Organ failure

Box 18.2 Commonly used drugs associated with delirium

High risk drugs	Medium risk drugs
Anticholinergics	Quinidine-like drugs
Dopamine agonists	Antihistamines
Opiates	Calcium channel-blocking drugs
Corticosteroids	Beta-blocking drugs
Tricyclic antidepressants	Benzodiazepines
Low potency antipsychotics	
Lithium	
Nonsteroidal anti-inflammatory drugs	
Digitalis	
Disopyramide	
Theophyline/aminophylline	

Derived from Karlsson (1999).

This list is not meant to be exhaustive and may under-represent drugs recently placed on the market. Of particular importance because of their frequency of use and their propensity for causing delirium are: anti-parkinsonian drugs, corticosteroid drugs, opiates, and cardiac drugs.

Anti-parkinsonian drugs

The drug treatment of Parkinson's disease (PD) is frequently complicated by the emergence of psychosis. The reasons are multifactorial but drug-induced states are common since the treatment of PD involves the two most common delirium-inducing classes of medication – anticholinergics and dopamine agonists. Neuropsychiatric symptoms secondary to drug treatment have been reported to vary from 5% to 17% in nondemented Parkinson's patients; however, the risk is much higher in the presence of dementia, with rates between 42% and 81% (Kuzuhara, 2001). In a study of 300 PD patients treated with anti-parkinsonian drugs, Chana et al (1994) reported visual hallucinations in 19%, confusion in 10%, and delusions in 6%. Self-report measures have suggested that the rate of drug-induced hallucinations may be as high as 26% in PD (Sanchez-Ramos et al, 1993). Visual hallucinations are the most common of these reactions and typically occur in clear consciousness but may also occur in the course of a delirium. The hallucinations are usually fully formed common images such as people, animals, and inanimate objects. The fact that they usually occur at night and are accompanied by vivid dreams and sleep disturbance may reflect a subclinical delirium picture. The perceptual abnormalities may have an illusory quality and are most often silent. Auditory and tactile hallucinations have been reported but appear to be rare. Delusions during the treatment of PD are typically persecutory in nature, with themes of physical threat, poisoning or being filmed/recorded, while delusions of jealousy have also been reported (Kuzuhara, 2001). Delusions are usually preceded by sleep disturbance, dreams, and visual hallucinations. The risk factors for developing psychosis during anti-parkinsonian treatment include: advanced age, dementia, premorbid psychiatric disturbance, and high doses of anti-parkinsonian drugs. Duration and severity of PD and duration of drug treatment are more controversial as risk factors.

All drugs used in the treament of PD have been implicated in the cause of psychosis. Levodopa, a dopamine synthesis precursor, first introduced in the 1970s, has become a cornerstone in the treatment of PD. Case reports of neuropsychiatric sequelae to levodopa therapy soon appeared and included descriptions of visual hallucinations, delusions, hypomania, and other syndromes (depression, anxiety, and hypersexuality) (Celesia and Barr, 1970; Jenkins and Groh, 1970). Early reports of controlled-release levodopa used for motor fluctuations and dyskinesias suggested no worsening of psychotic adverse events (Bush et al, 1989); however, this has been questioned, with reports of marked exacerbations of hallucinations and confusion following switches from standard levodopa treatment (Joseph et al, 1995). Dopamine agonists such as bromocriptine, pergolide, and apomorphine are usually used later in the course of illness. These agents are also associated with similar neuropsychiatric sequelae to those seen with levodopa such as visual hallucinations, persecutory delusions, and alterations to the conscious state (Lieberman et al, 1976; Stern et al, 1984; Stocchi et al, 1993). There appears to be a strong dose effect in causation of psychotic symptoms but little difference between agents in the propensity to cause neuropsychiatric symptoms (Young et al, 1997).

Anticholinergic drugs were among the first treatments for PD and continue to have a central role in treatment. These drugs are well known for neuropsychiatric effects in nonparkinsonian subjects including visual hallucinations and confusional states. Reports in PD patients have varied from 0% to 100% of patients (Young et al, 1997). The presence of dementia is particularly predisposing. The N-methyl-D-aspartate (NMDA) antagonists amantadine and memantine are second-line anti-parkinsonian drugs. As with the dopamine agonists and anticholinergic drugs, the NMDA antagonists are associated with emergence of visual hallucinations, which may occur in isolation or may be accompanied by signs of delirium or persecutory delusions (Harper and Knothe, 1973; Postma and van Tilburg, 1975). Short duration placebo-controlled studies of amantadine show no increased incidence of neuropsychiatric effects; however, longer-term studies suggest that the peak incidence is around the third to ninth month of treatment. While placebo-controlled trials of the monoamine oxidase B inhibitor, selegiline, suggest few significant neuropsychiatric adverse events in PD, Yahr et al (1983) reported hallucinations in 8% and confusion in 25% of 79 patients with advanced PD when selegeline was added to the existing treatment regime.

Corticosteroids

While the original report by Harvey Cushing on the effects of increased endogenous corticosteroids did not emphasize psychiatric sequelae (Cushing, 1932), more recent studies have suggested high rates of affective disorder. Cases of depression significantly outweigh those of elevated mood. 'Atypical' depression occurs in around half of those with Cushing's syndrome, while more typical major depression is seen in 12% of patients (Dorn et al, 1997). The first reports of psychiatric side effects to cortisone, an exogenous corticosteroid, appeared in the same year as its commercial release in 1950 (Boland and Headley, 1950; Soffer et al, 1950). The term 'steroid psychosis' was coined to describe the psychiatric sequelae; however, the features did not conform to a delirium picture and early case series reports included descriptions of patients with depression, dissociation, hypomania, and psychotic symptoms including persecutory delusions and hallucinations (Clark et al, 1952, 1953; Lewis and Fleminger, 1954). In an early case series reported by Rome and Braceland (1952), four major groups of responses were described including: (1) mild mood elevation/euphoria; (2) an effusive, expansive mood accompanied by restlessness and insomnia; (3) a mixed affective response characterized by marked anxiety and fluctuations of mood from lethargy, tearfulness and indifference to excitement and restlessness; and (4) 'grossly psychotic' reactions characterized by hallucinations, delusions, and marked mood variability. The first two groups accounted for 60% of the patients, the third group 25–30%, and the last group around 10%. While the reports of the incidence of psychiatric sequelae in uncontrolled studies vary from 1.6% to 62%, Lewis and Smith (1983) reported a weighted incidence of around 5.7%. This later review and case series concluded that, rather than a clearly definable steroid psychosis, patients could be grouped into two main groups: an affective group including mania and depression, which made up 75% of cases, and a toxic/organic group characterized by perplexity, disorientation, hallucinations, and delusions constituting the remaining 25% of cases. Manic episodes are more frequent than depressive episodes and are characterized by early symptoms of insomnia, distractability and excitability and later features of hyperactivity, euphoria, pressured speech, and irritability. Naber et al (1996) reported 13 cases of manic-like episodes of 50 patients receiving steroids compared with only five cases of depression. Corticosteroids may be responsible for up to 54% of cases of organic mania seen in general medical wards (Rundell and Wise, 1989). In a small series reported by Sharfstein et al (1982) there was a tendency for mania to emerge during corticosteroid treatment and for depressive symptoms to appear following discontinuation. The issue of delirium and psychosis remains a vexed one. Early studies did not report classical changes of disorientation and attention characteristic of delirium and there are case reports of psychotic symptoms emerging without attentional and cognitive change (Mullen and Romans-Clarkson, 1993).

The clinical course of psychiatric symptoms following commencement of steroids remains unclear. Lewis and Smith (1983) reported that 39–43% of patients experienced onset of symptoms in the first week, 57–62% within the first two weeks and 89–93% within the first six weeks. The median onset was around 11 days, which was slightly longer than the 5.9 days reported by Hall et al (1979). On closer inspection of the Lewis and Smith (1983) case series, there appears to be a bimodal distribution of cases with an early group occurring in the first week similar to that reported by Hall et al (1979) and a later cluster after three weeks of treatment. While the symptomatic profile does not appear to correlate with time to onset of symptoms, delirious and psychotic reactions are probably of short duration (less than one week), while affective episodes appear more prolonged – around three weeks for mania and perhaps longer for depression (Lewis and Smith, 1983). Complete recovery is the normal outcome.

Identification of risk factors for steroid psychosis is complex. Risk appears unrelated to age, past history of psychiatric illness or current medical illness for which steroids are administered. Marked female preponderance may be related to case series involving illnesses with underlying female over-representation such as systemic lupus erythematosus and rheumatoid arthritis; however, some female preponderance persisted after exclusion of these diseases. When the incidence of psychiatric syndromes is reported by gender, 19.7% of steroid-treated females developed a psychiatric syndrome compared with only 3.3% of males (p <0.001) (Lewis and Smith, 1983). The dosage of corticosteroid appears to be the strongest risk factor, with 1.3% having psychiatric reactions to steroids at doses of less than 40 mg equivalents of prednisolone per day, 4.6% at doses between 41 mg and 80 mg per day and 18.4% in those receiving more than 80 mg per day (Boston Collaborative Drug Surveillance Program, 1972). The mean dose of prednisolone among patients with psychiatric disturbance was 59.5 mg, significantly higher than mean dosages found with other adverse events such as gastrointestinal reactions (36.1 mg, p <0.05) or those without adverse reactions (33.1 mg, p <0.001) (Boston Collaborative Drug Surveillance Program, 1972). The dose-response effect could not be demonstrated for onset or duration of symptoms. Case reports suggest, however, that significant reactions can occur even at very low doses. Previous steroid-related psychiatric disturbance may not predict future episodes on re-exposure (Lewis and Smith, 1983).

Opiate-related psychoses

The majority of studies examining psychotic reactions to opiates have examined cancer patients frequently in palliative care wards. While opiates and dehydration are the most commonly reported causes of delirium in these populations, data suggest that the delirium is frequently multifactorial with a median of 3 (range 1–6) identified precipitating causes per episode of delirium (Lawler, 2002). This finding makes it difficult to be confident about specific opiate-related effects in these populations. Despite this, opiate-related neuropsychiatric syndromes have been identified including cognitive dysfunction, delirium, and organic hallucinosis. The most commonly studied neuropsychiatric syndrome seen with opiate use is cognitive dysfunction characterized by memory and concentration abnormalities. Cognitive dysfunction was found to occur in up to 77% of patients on brief testing over a seven-day period (Leipzig et al, 1987); however, rates were found to be lower on admission (20–44%) and higher before death (80–90%) (Lawler, 2002).

The more serious syndrome of delirium is less common during opiate administration. Leipzig et al (1987) reported that 19 of 35 (54%) patients with metastatic cancer admitted to a palliative care unit for pain control developed delirium. This figure is higher than that reported by Maddocks et al (1996) who studied 100 consecutive palliative care admissions of which 91 required opiate analgesia and 15 developed delirium (16%). The increased rate of delirium in the Leipzig et al (1987) cohort is most likely related to the focus on pain relief as the reason for admission and probable increased opiate use in these patients. There was a significant increase in delirium in patients over the age of 65 given opiates (69%) compared with those under 65 (38%) ($p = 0.02$), suggesting age as a vulnerability factor (Leipzig et al, 1987). While the duration of the delirium is unclear, the effect is usually short-lived. Bruera et al (1989) suggest that delirium is most common during escalation of dosing and resolution occurs relatively quickly. There appears to be a relationship to the type of opiate used. Morphine appears to be associated with delirium in up to 25% of terminally ill patients (Maddocks et al, 1996) while change of opiate or rotation of opiates has been reported to improve delirium (Bruera et al, 1995; Maddocks et al, 1996). Without well-controlled comparison studies, it is not yet possible to say which opiate is associated with least delirium; however, some data suggest that oxycodone and fentanyl may reduce the incidence (Kalso and Vainio, 1988; Caraceni et al, 1994). While visual hallucinations are the most common psychotic manifestation during opiate-induced delirium (Caraceni et al, 1994), case reports suggest that visual hallucinations without delirium may also occur during opiate administration. Bruera et al (1992) reported four cases of 55 cancer patients (7%) who developed isolated visual hallucinations while receiving hydromorphone subcutaneously or orally for pain relief. In three of these cases there was an associated sudden change in mood characterized by anxiety or depression. In all four cases the hallucinations responded rapidly to small doses of haloperidol (2 mg). Three of the four patients died in the following one to three weeks.

Cardiovascular drugs

Cardiovascular disease is associated with the greatest cause of death and disability in the developed world and the number of medical treatments developed for its treatment is constantly expanding. Neuropsychiatric syndromes associated with medical cardiovascular treatments are among the first described cases of drug-induced delirium and are increasingly important with the widespread use of modern treatments. Of historical interest are reports of mainly depressive reactions to drugs such as guanethidine, reserpine, and methyldopa. In this chapter we will cover more contemporary cardiovascular drugs with an emphasis on calcium channel blockers, class 1 antiarrhythmic agents, and angiotensin-converting enzyme (ACE) inhibitors.

Digoxin

The relationship between digitalis treatment and neuropsychiatric symptoms was first noted by William Withering (1785 in King, 1950) who reported that the 'brain is considerably affected'; however, he did not mention the syndrome of delirium, which was first raised by Duroziez (1874 in King, 1950) who coined the term 'deliere digitalique'. Preparations of digitalis during this period included tinctures, powdered/macerated leaf and the 'wine of Trousseau', which was administered to patients with a number of medical illnesses including nephritis, rheumatic fever, cirrhosis of the liver, and even delirium tremens (King, 1950). Duroziez reported 20 cases of digitalis complications including 13 cases of delirium. King (1950) added to the literature with six case reports of delirium associated with digitalis therapy, which was surprisingly still administered in the form of a powdered leaf or more regular preparations of digitoxin or lanatoside C. In each of these cases the delirium cleared with a reduction or cessation of the digitalis preparation and King concluded that, rather than cerebral circulatory change, the delirium was most likely due to intoxication with the drug.

There does not appear to be a specific digoxin delirium but rather a large number of presentations have been reported including affective change with manic-like symptoms of restlessness, irritability, insomnia, and euphoria, or a depressive-like syndrome of lethargy, fatigue, and appetite loss (see Keller and Frishman, 2003, for recent review). Delusions and hallucinations are also common. Digoxin plasma levels are routinely ordered when prescribing digoxin, to help guide the physician in maximizing therapeutic effect while minimizing toxicity. It appears that digoxin levels within the so-called therapeutic range do not prevent digoxin-induced delirium, as cases have been reported even within these restrictions (Eisendrath and Sweeney, 1987; Smith et al, 1992).

Calcium channel blockers

Calcium channel blockers are a heterogeneous group of medications commonly used in the treatment of hypertension, tachyarrhythmias, and ischemic heart disease. While there has been some interest in their use in the treatment of affective disorders, particularly mania, case reports suggest that they may also precipitate neuropsychiatric complications. Jacobsen et al (1987) reported the emergence of delirium with auditory, visual, and tactile hallucinations in a young woman who received verapamil for the treatment of her bipolar disorder. Fogelman (1988) also reported thought disorder and depressive symptoms in a 45-year-old man treated with verapamil for hypertension. A similar reaction has been reported with nifedipine (Ahmad, 1994) and there are at least three case reports of diltiazem-induced delirium characterized by either schizophreniform symptoms of auditory and visual hallucinations and paranoid delusions, depressive or manic symptoms (Palat and Movahed, 1986; Busche, 1988; Binder et al, 1991).

Class 1 antiarrhythmic agents

The antiarrhythmic drugs designated as class 1 are generally thought to act by blocking sodium channels. Cinchonism, a syndrome of quinidine toxicity, includes symptoms of delirium and confusion (Rollo, 1975). Case reports of hallucinations, persecutory delusions, and psychomotor agitation have also been described in patients taking quinidine below therapeutic levels (Deleu and Schmedding, 1987; Johnson et al, 1990). Saravay et al (1987) reported 15 patients with psychiatric complications of lignocaine treatment. The majority of patients had prominent anxiety and depressive symptoms, 53% had symptoms of delirium and 40% had perceptual abnormality including visual illusions and hallucinations. Neuropsychiatric syndromes have also been described with procainamide, disopyramide, tocainide, flecainide, and the class III agent amiodarone (see Keller and Frishman, 2003, for recent review).

Other cardiac drugs

A number of other medications used in treating cardiovascular disorders have been reported to induce delirium. ACE inhibitors are frequently prescribed for hypertension and cardiac failure. While there are some early reports of mood improvement on captopril (Zubenko and Nixon, 1984; Dieken, 1986), mania has also been reported in patients treated with captopril and lisinopril (Gajula and Berlin, 1993; Skop and Masterson, 1995). In contrast, an association with depression has been reported with enalopril and quinapril (Patterson, 1989; Gunduz et al, 1999) and case-controlled studies have suggested that ACE inhibitors may be more associated with depressive reactions than elevations of mood (Keller and Frishman, 2003). In addition to mood effects, ACE inhibitors have also been reported to cause delirium and visual hallucinations (Gillman and Sandyk, 1985; Haffner et al, 1993). Beta-adrenergic blockers, used widely in the treatment of hypertension and ischemic heart disease, are frequently considered to be depressogenic; however, these effects may be no more frequent than with other antihypertensive drugs. Keller and Frishman (2003) reviewed psychiatric disturbance associated with propranolol in 31 studies and found an incidence of hallucinations and illusions of 0.6%, and several case reports have associated atenolol with delirium.

Drug-induced disorders of water homeostasis

Electrolyte disturbances are a frequent cause of delirium in medically and psychiatrically treated patients. Thiazide diuretic drugs have been associated with delirium and, since they have very low penetration into the central nervous system (Seno et al, 1969), this is most likely secondary to electrolyte disturbances or the alteration of renal excretion of other drugs e.g. lithium (Siegel et al, 1998). One important and serious cause of iatrogenic-induced delirium is that of the drug-induced syndrome of inappropriate antidiuretic hormone secretion (SIADH). The reported incidence of hyponatremia secondary to SIADH ranges from 6.4% of long-term psychiatric inpatients to 11% of psychiatric patients admitted to an acute inpatient service (Siegel et al, 1998). The hyponatremia associated with SIADH commonly initially presents as delirium but may progress to seizures, coma, and death if not recognized. SIADH is caused by drug-induced release of ADH from the posterior pituitary or an enhancement of the action of ADH on renal collecting ducts. Psychotropic drugs are frequently implicated in SIADH, including phenothiazines, tricyclic antidepressants, monoamine oxidase inhibitors and selective serotonin reuptake inhibitors (SSRIs) (Siegel et al, 1998; Kirby and Ames, 2001; Kirby et al, 2002).

Serotonin and neuroleptic malignant syndromes

The use of psychotropic and related drugs in the treatment of mental symptoms can occasionally lead to psychotic syndromes. The two most severe of these are related to serotonergic agonist drugs (serotonin syndrome, SS) and dopamine-blocking drugs (neuroleptic malignant syndrome, NMS). While there are common features of these two syndromes there are also important differences. Both syndromes are associated with delirium-like features of disorientation, fluctuations of the conscious state, and hallucinations (Gillman, 1998). Also common to both syndromes are prominent sweating, pyrexia, tachypnea, and tachycardia. Gillman (1998) suggests that the most important feature differentiating SS from NMS is the presence of various manifestations of clonus and the presence of serotonergic agonist drugs. NMS, on the other hand, is characterized by motor features of rigidity, bradykinesia, mutism, and the presence of dopamine D2 receptor-blocking drugs. Whereas agitation can be an early manifestation of NMS, most cases proceed to bradykinesia, in contrast to SS where motor overactivity is the norm. A further conceptual difference is that NMS is perceived as an idiosyncratic response to dopamine-blocking drugs secondary to as yet ill-defined mechanisms, while SS appears to be an inevitable consequence of serotonergic toxicity since it can be reliably reproduced in animal models with excessive serotonergic activity (Gillman, 1998).

The history of SS suggests a significant role for drug interactions as being largely causative in humans. Perhaps the first description of SS in humans was that of Mitchell (1955) in a patient on a combination of iproniazid (which has monoamine oxidase inhibitor [MAOI] properties) and pethidine (which has serotonin reuptake inhibitor [SRI] properties). Multiple case reports have since appeared implicating combinations of MAOIs/tricyclic antidepressants, MAOIs/pethidine, and MAOIs/L-tryptophan (for reviews see Sternbach, 1991; Gillman, 1998). Since this time a dose-effect relationship has been shown in animals and humans, with increased fatalities occurring with more potent SRIs in combination with MAOIs. Monotherapy with SRIs, even in overdose, rarely results in SS (Gillman, 1998). Of importance, nonpsychotropic drugs with SRI activity have frequently been reported to be implicated in the development of SS, especially in combination with MAOIs and other SRIs and include 'over-the-counter' preparations of antihistamine drugs (e.g. chlorpheniramine), opiate analgesics (e.g. pethidine, tramadol), and anti-migraine drugs (sumatriptan and dihydroergotamine) (Gillman, 1998).

Nondrug-associated iatrogenic psychosis

Intensive care unit (ICU) delirium

The so-called 'intensive care unit (ICU) syndrome' and 'ICU psychosis' refers to a constellation of symptoms frequently seen in patients admitted to the ICU and is characterized by fluctuations of the conscious state, disorientation, delusions, hallucinations, and changes in behavior such as aggression or passivity. The onset is rapid and the duration is usually brief (one to two days) (McGuire et al, 2000). This presentation is consistent with classical delirium and there appear to be no distinctive features to justify an alternative label. The usual causes of delirium need to be excluded; however, the apparent increased risk of delirium in the ICU most probably relates to pathophysiologic changes of severe illness, postoperative metabolic disturbances, the increased use of often toxic drugs, and the severity of the underlying illness. Early research suggested a unique role of sleep deprivation in the ICU with constant lighting and activity that was proposed to disturb the normal circadian rhythms of the patient (Kornfield et al, 1965). At this time there is no clear evidence to support a role for sleep deprivation as a cause for delirium occurring in the ICU (McGuire et al, 2000).

Postoperative delirium

The postoperative period is a frequent time for the emergence of delirium. The incidence varies markedly according to the study, the type of operation, patient demographics, and the underlying pathology, but overall appears to be around 37% (Dyer et al, 1995). As with the ICU syndrome, there do not appear to be distinctive features of the 'postoperative delirium' and the cause is frequently multifactorial. Particular attention should be paid to postoperative metabolic disturbance including electrolytes, blood gases and blood glucose, pain, infection, blood loss and undiagnosed organ damage such as the heart (infarction), brain (stroke), lungs (embolus) and kidneys (failure). A number of highly deliriogenic drugs are frequently used in the postoperative period, which may contribute to the incidence of delirium following operation and include opiate analgesia and some antibiotics. Fluid balance should be carefully attended to in the postoperative period. Pre-existing conditions may predispose to postoperative delirium and should be thoroughly assessed before theatre if possible, including PD and dementia. Some surgical procedures are also of particular risk including long duration procedures, cardiac surgery (hypoxia), orthopedic surgery (fat emboli), and cataract surgery with loss of vision and the administration of powerful anticholinergic drugs (for review see Winawer, 2001).

Etiology of iatrogenic psychosis

Aging is associated with a decline in physiological function. The various physiological changes are well recognized and have been described in detail (Salzman et al, 1988; Troen, 2003). These physiological changes lead to alterations in both the pharmacokinetics and pharmacodynamics of medications (Crooks et al, 1976; Vestal, 1978; Greenblatt et al, 1982; Swift, 1990; Turnheim, 2003). In general it can be stated that aging leads to both an increased variability in drug kinetics and an increased susceptibility to the effects (both desired and unwanted) of drugs compared with younger adults.

Physiological changes of aging

A reduction in homeostatic capacities with the aging process is fundamental to senescence but the decline in functional reserve varies considerably between individuals (Troen, 2003; Turnheim, 2003). Loss of skeletal muscle and various endocrine and immune function changes result in frailty in the very old (Walston and Fried, 1999). As a consequence the elderly are increasingly prone to disease. In general there is a loss of efficiency with increasing age of physiological functions. Important changes have been described for the cardiovascular system. In addition to the anatomic and histologic changes, decreased cardiac output and stroke volume, increased blood pressure and peripheral vascular resistance are also noted (Montoye et al, 1968). In the central nervous system there is an increase in neurofibrillary tangles and senile plaques (in the absence of Alzheimer's disease), as well as changes in neurotransmitters and their synthetic enzyme systems (Davidson, 1978; Bartus et al, 1982). Changes also occur in the respiratory system where there is a steady decline in arterial pO_2, maximum O_2 consumption, and lung volume (Ritschel, 1988). The gastric mucosa and liver are affected by aging, resulting in a number of important changes. In particular there is an increase in gastric pH, a decrease in hepatic oxidation capacity with the decline in activity of hepatic cytochrome P450 enzymes (Bender, 1968; O'Malley et al, 1971; Woodhouse and James, 1990). Even in the absence of renal disease there is a decline in renal function with aging. Age-dependent decreases in glomerular filtration have been demonstrated by the measurement of inulin or creatinine clearance (Friedman et al, 1972). Other physiologic changes evident with aging are changes in body composition. There is reduced lean body mass and body water, and an increase in fat tissue (Edelman and Liebman, 1959; Forbes and Reina, 1970). These latter changes have important effects on the pharmacokinetics of drugs with aging, resulting in decreased clearances and increased volumes of distribution (Crooks et al, 1976; Vestal, 1978; Greenblatt et al, 1982; Ritschel, 1988; Salzman et al, 1988).

A further potential physiological change with aging is in the permeability of the blood–brain barrier (BBB) to drugs and infectious agents (Neuwelt, 2004). The BBB isolates the extracellular fluid of the brain from the general circulation. It consists of a layer of endothelial cells that line the cerebral vascular beds and restrict the passage of soluble molecules (Golden and Pollack, 2003; Neuwelt, 2004). The BBB permeability of the majority of molecules is predicted by their lipid solubility – only the unbound fraction of lipophilic substances or molecules for which specific transport processes exist can penetrate the brain (Neuwelt, 2004). Recent studies show that this passive model of the BBB does not fully explain the limited penetration of many lipid-soluble molecules (Neuwelt, 2004). Rather the process is more dynamic: some small solutes with high octanol/water partition coefficients poorly penetrate the BBB. These substances are actively transported back into the blood by efflux systems such as P-glycoprotein and glutathione-dependent multidrug resistance-associated proteins (Golden and Pollack, 2003). The effect of aging on these proteins is not known but clearly alterations would affect the permeability of the central nervous system to drugs or other agents (e.g. infectious agents).

Pharmacodynamic changes of aging

Alterations in neurotransmitter concentrations and the number of their associated receptor subtypes vary according to brain region (Sheldon, 1963). Furthermore, although the number of receptors may change there can be compensatory changes in their sensitivity. Reduced activity of the enzyme choline acetyl transferase, responsible for the production of acetylcholine and the associated changes in cholinergic receptors, is believed to be responsible for memory difficulties with aging (Bartus et al, 1982). In particular changes in cholinergic receptors in the hippocampus are believed to be pivotal in the memory difficulties associated with Alzheimer's disease. Changes in other neurotransmitter systems, particularly serotonin and noradrenaline, may contribute to the etiology of depression in the elderly (Salzman, 1984).

Advancing age has been shown to increase the number of corrective movements necessary to stand upright (Sheldon, 1963). This in turn has been related to a reduced number of dopamine D2 receptors in the striatum. Increased sensitivity to postural hypotension induced by drugs with adrenoreceptor-blocking effects has been related to changes in the baroreceptors in the carotid sinus and elsewhere (Caird et al, 1973).

Changes in neurotransmitter receptors may also account, at least in part, for the increased susceptibility of the elderly to the effects of medication. For example, the increased sensitivity of the elderly to the postural and sedative effects of benzodiazepines has been related to an increased density and sensitivity of benzodiazepine binding sites in the aging central nervous system (Castelden et al, 1977; Campbell and Somerton, 1982). Similarly the elderly are more vulnerable to the anticholinergic effects of antipsychotic and antidepressant medication (Salzman, 1984). Changes in dopamine receptor sensitivity with aging may also account for the higher incidence and greater severity of extrapyramidal side effects of antipsychotic drugs in the elderly (Salzman, 1984). The elderly may also be less sensitive to the effects of beta-adrenergic receptor agonists and antagonists than younger subjects (Vestal et al, 1979; Swift, 1990).

Possible pharmacodynamic mechanisms in iatrogenic psychosis

Most reviews of medication-induced psychosis conclude that a large number of drugs may cause delirium in susceptible individuals; however, it is possible to identify some commonalities of action of drugs at high risk of doing so. The most studied of these imply an important role for the neurotransmitters acetylcholine, dopamine, and serotonin. Anticholinergic drugs acting at muscarinic receptors may reproduce many of the cardinal features of delirium including attentional and learning deficits, hallucinations, hyperactivity, and slowing of the electroencephalogram (EEG). A large number of drugs with anti-cholinergic activity have been found to cause delirium (for review see Trzepacz, 2000) and studies have shown that serum anticholinergic activity positively correlates with delirium in elderly hospitalized medical inpatients, delirious post-cardiotomy patients, post-electroconvulsive therapy confusional states, and patients with delirium in the ICU (for review see Tune, 2000). These findings may also explain the vulnerability of patients with dementia in which there is loss of cholinergic cell bodies, with increased rates of delirium (Tune, 2000). Furthermore, acetylcholinesterase inhibitor drugs have been shown to reverse anticholinergic drug-induced delirium (Trzepacz, 2000).

As is the case with anticholinergic drugs, dopamine agonist drugs such as L-dopa, bupropion, and cocaine have been reported to cause delirium, and produce slowing of the EEG typical of delirium. Stimulation of different dopamine receptor subtypes results in opposite effects on motor activity and it has been suggested that this may explain the hyperactivity, hypoactivity or mixed motor activity picture seen in patients with delirium (Trzepacz, 2000). In addition, there is a complex interaction between dopamine and acetyl-choline neurotransmitters in the brain so that manipulation of one system may reverse a delirium caused by abnormalities in the other, e.g. chlorpro-mazine and tacrine may both reverse anticholinergic drug-induced delirium (Itil and Fink, 1966). Serotonergic mechanisms have also been hypothesized in the etiology of delirium (see SS above) and serotonergic agents have been shown to increase prefrontal dopamine release (Tanda et al, 1994). Furthermore, lowered plasma serotonin and serotonin precursor (tryptophan) have been reported in delirious patients post-cardiotomy (van der Mast and Fekkes, 2000). Other endogenous substances implicated in the etiology of drug-induced delirium include the neurotransmitter systems GABA (γ amino butyric acid), glutamate/NMDA (N-methyl-D-aspartate), noradrenaline, the substrates of the HPA (hypothalamic pituitary adrenal) axis, and immunological proteins.

Conclusion

Iatrogenic psychoses are more commonly classified as either delirium or substance-induced psychosis in modern nomenclature. They are a group of very common and potentially dangerous syndromes occurring particularly in the elderly. Frequently the 'iatrogenic psychoses' occur as a consequence of commonly used medications but most often the cause is multifactorial and contributions from other sources need to be assessed, e.g. infection, electrolyte disturbances. Commonly used drugs may precipitate the syndrome through direct effects on targeted receptor systems, direct effects on nontargeted receptor systems or indirect effects. The changing physiology of the elderly may explain the preponderance of delirium in this group; however, underlying pathological processes such as dementia and general medical illness also need consideration.

References

Ahmad S, Nifedipine-induced acute psychosis, *J Am Geriatr Soc* (1994) **32**:408.

American Pyschiatric Association, *Diagnostic and Statistical Manual of Mental Disorders*, 4th edn (DSM-IV) (American Psychiatric Association: Washington, DC, 1994).

Bartus RT, Dean RLI, Beer B, The cholinergic hypothesis of geriatric memory dysfunction, *Science* (1982) **217**:408–17.

Bender AD, Effect of age on intestinal absorption: implications for drug absorption in the elderly, *J Am Geriatr Soc* (1968) **16**:1331–9.

Binder EF, Cayabyab L, Ritchie DJ, Birge SJ, Diltiazem-induced psychosis and a possible diltiazem-lithium interaction, *Arch Intern Med* (1991) **151**:373–4.

Boland EW, Headley NE, Management of rheumatoid arthritis with smaller (maintenance) doses of cortisone acetate, *JAMA* (1950) **144**:365.

Boston Collaborative Drug Surveillance Program, Acute adverse reactions to prednisolone in relation to dosage, *Clin Pharmacol Ther* (1972) **13**:694–8.

Bruera E, MacMillan K, Hansen J, The cognitive effects of the administration of narcotic analgesics in patients with cancer pain, *Pain* (1989) **39**:13–16.

Bruera E, Franco JJ, Maltoni M et al, Changing pattern of agitated impaired mental status in patients with advanced cancer: association with cognitive monitoring, hydration and opioid rotation, *J Pain Symptom Manage* (1995) **10**:287–91.

Bruera E, Schoeller T, Montejo G, Organic hallucinosis in patients receiving high doses of opiates for cancer pain, *Pain* (1992) **48**:397–9.

Bucht G, Gustafson Y, Sandberg O, Epidemiology of delirium, *Dement Geriatr Cogn Disord* (1999) **10**:315–18.

Busche CJ, Organic psychosis caused by diltiazem, *J Roy Soc Med* (1988) **81**:296–7.

Bush DF, Liss CL, Morton A, An open, multicenter, longterm treatment evaluation on Sinemet CR, *Neurology* (1989) **39** (Suppl 2):101–4.

Caird FI, Andrews JR, Kennedy RD, Effect of posture on blood pressure in the elderly, *Br Heart J* (1973) **35**:527–30.

Campbell AJ, Somerton DT, Benzodiazepine drug effects on body sway in elderly subjects, *J Clin Exp Gerontol* (1982) **4**:341–7.

Caraceni A, Martini C, De Conno F, Ventafridda V, Organic brain syndromes and opioid administration for cancer pain, *J Pain Symptom Manage* (1994) **9**:527–33.

Castleden CM, George CF, Marcer D, Hallett C, Increased sensitivity to nitrazepam in old age, *BMJ* (1977) **1**:10–12.

Celesia GG, Barr AN, Psychosis and other psychiatric manifestations of levodopa therapy, *Arch Neurol* (1970) **23**:193–200.

Chana P, Weiser R, Jimenez J, Origin of psychiatric complications in Parkinson's disease, *Mov Disord* (1994) **9** (Suppl 1):59.

Clark LD, Bauer W, Cobb S, Preliminary observations on mental disturbance occurring in patients under therapy with cortisone and ACTH, *N Engl J Med* (1952) **246**:205–16.

Clark LD, Quarton GC, Cobb S, Bauer W, Further observations on mental disturbances associated with cortisone and ACTH therapy, *N Engl J Med* (1953) **249**:178–83.

Crooks J, O'Malley K, Stevenson IH, Pharmacokinetics in the elderly, *Clin Pharmacokinet* (1976) **1**:280–96.

Cushing H, The basophil adenomas of the pituitary body and their clinical manifestations (pituitary basophilism), *Bulletin of Johns Hopkins Hospital* (1932) **50**:137–95.

Davidson AN, Biochemical aspects of the aging brain, *Age Ageing* (1978) **7** (Suppl):4–11.

Deleu D, Schmedding E, Acute psychosis as idiosyncratic reaction to quinidine: report of two cases, *BMJ* (1987) **294**:1001–2.

Dieken RF, Captopril treatment of depression, *Biol Psych* (1986) **21**:1425–8.

Dorn LD, Burgess ES, Friedman TC et al, The longitudinal course of psychopathology in Cushing's Syndrome after correction of hypercortisolism, *J Clin Endocr Metab* (1997) **82**:912–19.

Dyer CB, Ashton CM, Teasedale TA, Postoperative delirium, *Arch Intern Med* (1995) **155**:461–5.

Edelman IS, Liebman J, Anatomy of body water and electrolytes, *Am J Med* (1959) **27**:256–77.

Eisendrath SJ, Sweeney MA, Toxic neuropsychiatric effects of digoxin at therapeutic serum concentrations, *Am J Psychiatry* (1987) **144**:506–7.

Fogelman J, Verapamil caused depression, confusion and impotence, *Am J Psychiatry* (1988) **145**:380.

Forbes GR, Reina JC, Adult lean body mass declines with age: some longitudinal observations, *Metabolism* (1970) **19**:653–63.

Francis J, Martin D, Kapoor WN, A prospective study of delirium in hospitalized elderly, *JAMA* (1990) **263**:1097–101.

Friedman SA, Raizner AE, Rosen H et al, Functional defects in the aging kidney, *Ann Intern Med* (1972) **76**:42–5.

Gajula RP, Berlin RM, Captopril induced mania, *Am J Psychiatry* (1993) **150**:1429–30.

Gillman MA, Sandyk R, Reversal of captopril-induced psychosis with naloxone, *Am J Psychiatry* (1985) **142**:270.

Gillman PK, Serotonin syndrome: history and risk, *Fundam Clin Pharmacol* (1998) **12**:482–91.

Golden PL, Pollack GM, Blood-brain barrier efflux transport, *J Pharm Sci* (2003) **92**:1739–53.

Greenblatt DJ, Sellers EM, Shader RI, Drug disposition in old age, *N Engl J Med* (1982) **306**:1081–8.

Gunduz H, Georges JL, Fleishman S, Quinapril and depression, *Am J Psychiatry* (1999) **156**:114–5.

Haffner CA, Smith BS, Pepper C, Hallucinations as an adverse effect of angiotensin converting enzyme inhibition, *Postgrad Med J* (1993) **69**:240.

Hall RCW, Popkin MK, Stickney SK, Gardner ER, Presentation of steroid psychoses, *J Nerv Ment Dis* (1979) **167**:229–36.

Harper RW, Knothe BUC, Coloured Lilliputian hallucinations with amantadine, *Med J Aust* (1973) **1**:444–5.

Itil T, Fink M, Anticholinergic drug induced delirium: experimental modification, quantitative EEG and behavioural correlations, *J Nerv Ment Dis* (1966) **143**: 492–507.

Jacobsen FM, Sack DA, James SP, Delirium induced by verapamil, *Am J Psychiatry* (1987) **144**:248–52.

Jenkins RB, Groh RH, Mental symptoms in Parkinsonian patients treated with L-dopa, *Lancet* (1970) **11**:177–80.

Johnson AG, Day RO, Seldom WA, A functional psychosis precipitated by quinidine, *Med J Aust* (1990) **153**:47–9.

Joseph CL, Siple J, McWhorter K, Camicioli R, Adverse reactions to controlled release levodopa/carbidopa in older persons: case reports, *J Am Geriatr Soc* (1995) **43**:47–50.

Kalso E, Vainio A, Hallucinations during morphine but not during oxycodone treatment, *Lancet* (1988) **56**:912.

Karlsson I, Drugs that induce delirium, *Dement Geriatr Cogn Disord* (1999) **10**:412–15.

Keller S, Frishman WH, Neuropsychiatric effects of cardiovascular drug therapy, *Cardiol Rev* (2003) **11**:73–93.

King JT, Digitalis delirium, *Ann Intern Med* (1950) **33**:1360–72.

Kirby D, Ames D, Hyponatraemia and selective serotonin uptake inhibitors in elderly patients, *Int J Geriatr Psychiatry* (2001) **16**:484–93.

Kirby D, Harrigan S, Ames D, Hyponatraemia in elderly psychiatric patients treated with Selective Serotonin Reuptake Inhibitors and venlafaxine: a retrospective controlled study in an inpatient unit, *Int J Geriatr Psychiatry* (2002) **17**:231–7.

Kornfield DS, Zinberg S, Malm J, Psychiatric complications of open heart surgery, *N Engl J Med* (1965) **273**:287–9.

Kuzuhara S, Drug-induced psychotic symptoms in Parkinson's disease: problems, management and dilemma, *J Neurol* (2001) **248** (Suppl 3):28–31.

Lawler PG, The panorama of opioid-related cognitive dysfunction in patients with cancer: a critical literature appraisal, *Cancer* (2002) **94**:1836–53.

Leipzig RM, Goodman H, Gray G et al, Reversible, narcotic-associated mental status impairment in patients with metastatic cancer, *Pharmacology* (1987) **35**:47–54.

Lewis A, Fleminger JJ, The psychiatric risk from corticotrophin and cortisone, *Lancet* (1954) **1**:383–6.

Lewis DA, Smith RE, Steroid-induced psychiatric syndromes: a report of 14 cases and a review of the literature, *J Affect Disord* (1983) **5**:319–32.

Lieberman A, Kupersmith M, Estey E, Goldstein M, Treatment of Parkinson's disease with bromocriptine, *N Engl J Med* (1976) **295**:1400–4.

McGuire BE, Basten CJ, Ryan CJ, Gallagher J, Intensive care unit syndrome: a dangerous misnomer, *Arch Intern Med* (2000) **160**:906–9.

Maddocks I, Somogyi A, Abbott F et al, Attenuation of morphine-induced delirium in palliative care by substitution with infusion of oxycodone, *J Pain Symptom Manage* (1996) **12**:182–9.

Mitchell RS, Fatal toxic encephalitis occurring during iproniazid therapy in pulmonary tuberculosis, *Ann Intern Med* (1955) **42**:417–24.

Montoye HJ, Willis PW, Cunningham DA, Heart rate response to sub-maximal exercise: relation to age and sex, *J Gerontol* (1968) **23**:127–33.

Moore AR, O'Keefe ST, Drug-induced cognitive impairment in the elderly, *Drugs Aging* (1999) **15**:15–28.

Mullen RS, Romans-Clarkson SE, Behavioural sensitization and steroid-induced psychosis, *Br J Psychiatry* (1993) **162**:549–51.

Naber D, Sand P, Heigl B, Psychopathological and neuropsychological effects of 8-days corticosteroid treatment: a prospective study, *Psychoneuroendocrinology* (1996) **21**:25–31.

Neuwelt EA, Mechanism of disease: the blood brain barrier, *Neurosurgery* (2004) **54**:131–42.

O'Keefe S, Lavan J, The prognostic significance of delirium in older hospitalised patients, *J Am Geriatr Soc* (1997) **45**:174–8.

O'Malley K, Crooks J, Duke E, Stevenson IH, Effect of age and sex on human drug metabolism, *BMJ* (1971) **3**:607–9.

Palat GK, Movahed A, Secondary mania associated with diltiazem, *Clin Cardiol* (1986) **9**:39.

Patterson JF, Depression associated with enalapril, *South Med J* (1989) **82**:402–3.

Postma JU, van Tilburg W, Visual hallucinations and delirium during treatment with amantadine (Symmetrel), *J Am Geriatr Soc* (1975) **23**:212–5.

Ritschel WA, *Gerontokinetics: The Pharmacokinetics of Drugs in the Elderly* (Telford Press: New Jersey, 1988).

Rollo IM, Drugs used in the chemotherapy of malaria. In: Goodman LS, Gilman A, eds, *The Pharmacological Basis of Therapeutics*, 5th edn (Macmillan Publishing: New York, 1975).

Rome HP, Braceland FJ, The psychological response to ACTH, cortisone, hydrocortisone and related steroid substances, *Am J Psychiatry* (1952) **108**:641–51.

Rundell JR, Wise MG, Causes of organic mood disorder, *J Neuropsychiatry Clin Neurosci* (1989) **1**:398–400.

Salzman C, Neurotransmission in the aging central nervous system. In: Salzman C, ed, *Clinical Geriatric Psychopharmacology* (McGraw-Hill: New York, 1984) 18–31.

Salzman C, Satlin A, Burrows AB, Geriatric psychopharmacology. In: Schatzberg AF, Nemeroff CB, eds, *The American Psychiatric Association Press Textbook of Psychopharmacology*, 2nd edn (American Psychiatric Association: Washington, 1988) 961–77.

Sanchez-Ramos JR, Ortoll R, Singer C et al, Visual hallucinations in Parkinson's disease, *Ann Neurol* (1993) **34**:264–5.

Saravay SM, Marke J, Steinberg MD, Rabiner CJ, 'Doom anxiety' and delirium in lidocaine toxicity, *Am J Psychiatry* (1987) **144**:159–63.

Seno S, Shaw SM, Christian FE, Distribution and urinary excretion of frusemide in the rat, *J Pharmacol Sci* (1969) **58**:935–8.

Sharfstein SS, Sack DS, Fauci AS, Relationship between alternate-day corticosteroid therapy and behavioral abnormalities, *JAMA* (1982) **248**:2987–9.

Sheldon JH, The effects of age on the control of sway, *Gerontology* (1963) **5**:129–38.

Siegel AJ, Baldessarini RJ, Klepser MB et al, Primary and drug-induced disorders of water homeostasis in psychiatric patients: principles of diagnosis and management, *Harvard Rev Psychiatry* (1998) **6**:190–200.

Skop BP, Masterson BJ, Mania secondary to lisinopril therapy, *Psychosomatics* (1995) **36**:508–9.

Smith H, Janz TG, Erker M, Digoxin toxicity presenting as altered mental status in a patient with severe obstructive lung disease, *Heart Lung* (1992) **21**:78–80.

Soffer LJ, Levitt MF, Baehr G, Use of cortisone and adrenocorticotrophic hormone in acute disseminated lupus erythematosus, *Arch Intern Med* (1950) **86**:558–73.

Stern Y, Mayeux R, Ilson J et al, Pergolide therapy for Parkinson's disease: neurobehavioral changes, *Neurology* (1984) **34**:201–4.

Sternbach H, The serotonin syndrome, *Am J Psychiatry* (1991) **148**:705–13.

Stocchi F, Bramante L, Monge A et al, Apomorphine and lisuride infusion: a comparative chronic study, *Adv Neurol* (1993) **60**:653–5.

Swift GC, Pharmacodynamics: changes in homeostatic mechanisms, receptor and target organ sensitivity in the elderly, *Br Med Bull* (1990) **46**:36–52.

Tanda G, Carboni E, Frau R, DiChiari E, Increase in extracellular dopamine in the PFC: a trait of drugs with antidepressant potential?, *Psychopharmacology* (1994) **115**:285–8.

Troen BR, The biology of aging, *Mt Sinai J Med* (2003) **70**:3–22.

Trzepacz PT, Is there a final common neural pathway in delirium? Focus on acetylcholine and dopamine, *Semin Clin Neuropsychiatry* (2000) **5**:132–48.

Tune LE, Serum anticholinergic activity levels and delirium in the elderly, *Semin Clin Neuropsychiatry* (2000) **5**:149–53.

Turnheim K, When drug therapy gets old: pharmacokinetics and pharmacodynamics in the elderly, *Exp Gerontol* (2003) **38**:843–53.

van der Mast RC, Fekkes D, Serotonin and amino acids: partners in delirium pathophysiology?, *Semin Clin Neuropsychiatry* (2000) **5**:125–31.

Vestal RE, Drug use in the elderly: a review of problems and special considerations, *Drugs* (1978) **16**:358–82.

Vestal RE, Wood AJJ, Shand DG, Reduced β-adrenoceptor sensitivity in the elderly, *Clin Pharm Ther* (1979) **26**:181–6.

Walston J, Fried LP, Frailty and the older man, *Med Clin North Am* (1999) **83**:1173–94.

Winawer N, Postoperative delirium, *Med Clin North Amer* (2001) **85**:1229–39.

Woodhouse KW, James OFW, Hepatic drug metabolism and ageing, *Br Med Bull* (1990) **46**:22–35.

World Health Organization, *The ICD-10 Classification of Mental and Behavioural Disorders: Diagnostic Criteria for Research* (World Health Organization: Geneva, 1992).

Yahr MD, Mendoza MR, Moros D, Bergman KJ, Treatment of Parkinson's disease in early and late phases: use of pharmacological agents with special reference to deprenyl (selegeline), *Acta Neurol Scand* (1983) **68** (Suppl 95):95–102.

Young BK, Camicioli R, Ganzini L, Neuropsychiatric adverse effects of antiparkinsonian drugs: characteristics, evaluation and treatment, *Drugs Aging* (1997) **10**:367–83.

Zubenko GS, Nixon RA, Mood elevating effects of captopril in depressed patients, *Am J Psychiatry* (1984) **141**:110–11.

chapter 19

Conclusion: directions for future research and practice

Anne Hassett, David Ames and Edmond Chiu

In this concluding chapter the editors review the 18 previous chapters and consider the implications for clinical practice and further research.

In the first chapter on the historical background, Seeman and Jeste make clear that having reconceptualized schizophrenia through the Leeds Castle Consensus, we now have a new and viable framework for future research. The reworking of the phenomenology, etiological and risk factors, course and prognosis, and response to treatment, in the setting of early-onset schizophrenia (EOS), late-onset schizophrenia (LOS), and very-late-onset schizophrenia-like psychosis (VLOSLP) will provide many new opportunities for researchers and should lead to a much better understanding of the spectrum of schizophrenic disorders across the lifespan.

In Chapter 2 Hassett examines the thorny problem of defining psychotic disorders in an aging population. The phenomenology of negative symptoms and their relationship to cognitive impairment in EOS has a very important link to our understanding of LOS. How can negative symptoms be separated from cognitive impairment? Is cognitive impairment a necessary part of schizophrenia, a risk factor for its development or part of its pathology? Does the successful treatment (when available) of negative symptoms have the potential to restore the patient to full cognitive function? In this context, can the cholinesterase inhibitors be useful in the treatment of negative symptoms as well as for cognitive impairment in dementia? Some of the curious differences between LOS and EOS demand further clarification. Why do LOS and VLOSLP patients have far less (if any!) thought disorder and fewer negative symptoms? Can these phenomena assist the delivery of useful interventions?

The curious phenomenon of 'partition delusions' also seems to be more or less exclusive to VLOSLP. These three differences have raised the questions of whether LOS/VLOSLP and EOS have different etiologies or if age-related factors are adequate to explain such differences. The 'overlapping pathophysical pathways' suggested by Förstl et al (1994) would warrant exploration to address these questions.

Castle's review of the epidemiology of LOS (Chapter 3) shows it to be an area beset by methodological problems, including changing nomenclature, varying age cut-offs to designate 'late-onset', varying diagnostic criteria, and heterogeneity among clinical samples, particularly with regard to the overlap with subjects who may be dementing. The International Consensus Statement (Howard et al, 2000) recommended that a distinction be made between cases of schizophrenia-like psychosis with an onset between 40 and 60 years from those with an onset after the age of 60. Studies are now required to test the utility of this age-dependent separation, and to examine the role of proposed risk factors (genetic vulnerability, sex, cerebrovascular changes), and whether these exert differing levels of influence at particular life stages.

Alzheimer was hired by Kraepelin to find the lesions responsible for schizophrenia. In Chapter 4 Walterfang and colleagues indicate how much further modern imaging techniques have moved us towards that goal a century later. The answer seems to be 'a bit'. Despite some advances, studies using modern equipment are still bedevilled by nonrepresentative patient selection, confounding of results by medication effects, and the ubiquity of some potentially causative changes (e.g. white matter hyperintensities) in elderly subjects who do not have schizophrenia or related psychoses. At least these techniques are relatively noninvasive, but before applying an array of yet more powerful and costly imaging systems to populations of elderly people affected by psychotic phenomena, researchers might do well to take a step back and first ensure that the questions they are asking are likely to have heuristic utility and that the populations to be examined are representative of the disorder to be studied. In no other area of medicine is the maxim 'less is more' of such potential relevance as in imaging studies of psychoses occurring in late life.

Although LOS/VLOSLP frequently is associated with a pattern of generalized cognitive impairment, this does not appear to differ significantly from the cognitive profile of older persons with long-standing EOS. In Chapter 5 Almeida indicates that as research to date has only addressed this question indirectly, specific comparative studies between these two patient groups are required. Available evidence suggests that the cognitive deficits of EOS are not progressive in nature, whereas the long-term outcome for LOS remains unclear. At this stage we have only observational evidence to show that the onset of delusions and hallucinations in later life appears to be associated with the subsequent development of dementia, as with late-onset depression. On the other hand, the two small studies in this area did not find Alzheimer-like neuropathological changes in the brains of patients with LOS.

Although we need to understand the etiologies of LOS and VLOSLP much better, we still need to do what we can to help existing patients who are affected by these conditions now. In Chapter 6 Ritchie makes the very relevant point that there is no specific licencing requirement for a new antipsychotic drug to be tested in the elderly, either for the purposes of initial licencing or for later use. Including the elderly would increase the heterogeneity of trial samples, but unfortunately, subsequent well-designed trials have been very limited in number and scope. Prescribing for the elderly therefore relies to an unacceptable degree upon extrapolation from the much larger evidence base accumulated from the use of antipsychotic agents in younger populations with schizophrenia. There are several reasons to support more trials, which recruit elderly subjects with EOS, LOS, and VLOSLP; in particular, pharmacokinetic and pharmacodynamic changes in the elderly, co-morbid medical problems, and the greater likelihood of older patients being subject to the perils of polypharmacy are cogent arguments in this regard.

Psychosocial rehabilitation, through the re-setting of the World Health Organization (WHO) concepts of disability now seen as 'components of health' rather than 'consequences of disease', and the emphasis on function and participation, present the field with a fresh framework for the development of effective psychosocial rehabilitation interventions for the elderly with psychosis, as Camus and Mendonça-Lima indicate in Chapter 7. The inclusion of psychological strategies in the community-based multidisciplinary framework should be actively explored and tested. The translation from specialist programs to 'real world' clinical practice reality will challenge all old age psychiatry practitioners.

In Chapter 8, Kelleher and colleagues define multidisciplinary community-based long-term care as consisting of a range of specialized services, which are coordinated by a mental health clinician, usually a 'case manager', with the overall goal being to maximize an older person's ability to live independently in the community. For elderly patients with schizophrenia this is likely to include a range of management interventions across the biopsychosocial spectrum. This is a poorly researched area, which requires the application of stringent evidence-based practice in order to channel resources most appropriately and efficiently, and strengthen the models of rehabilitation as they apply to older patients with functional psychiatric disorders, such as schizophrenia. Activities of daily living assessments, housing advocacy, residential care assessments, carer issues, legal issues, community integration, and liaison with other relevant health and welfare providers are aspects of multidisciplinary community-based long-term care which need to be examined and evaluated as to their pertinence as 'core business' for clinicians.

Many now elderly people who developed schizophrenia in early adulthood spent much of their adult lives in large psychiatric institutions, later moving to their smaller successors such as rooming houses, hostels, and nursing homes. These individuals often have no or very limited experience of independent living and it is a challenging task to empower them and help them to fit back into communities they left half a century earlier. In Chapter 9 McDougall and Rota address the needs of this disenfranchized cohort. As they imply, the fact that previous accommodation and care have been suboptimal for most of these people is no reason to deny them the best we can offer in their later years.

As the World Psychiatric Association has set de-stigmatization as its priority for action, the double jeopardy of stigmatization towards the elderly and people with psychosis will demand effective de-stigmatization strategies from all who are working with this group of patients. Lindesay reviews this topic in Chapter 10. What then are effective strategies? Will public education, in any form, be useful; or will this rebound on those who are most vulnerable? In a broader sense, how well do we combat the 'agism' which is so pervasive? Will the establishment of quality mental health services for the elderly and achieving world best practice, be a vehicle to successful de-stigmatization?

Although delirium is one of the commonest causes of psychosis, there is still distressingly little known about the nature and course of the perceptual and delusional phenomena that delirious patients find so distressing. Cross-sectional studies usually have focused on the rates of psychotic symptoms, and post-delirium studies are reliant on the subject's capacity to recall their experiences during a delirious episode. In Chapter 11 Bhat highlights that future research needs to examine the relationship between the diversity of psychotic symptoms noted in patients with delirium and possible etiological factors. The diagnostic dilemma that arises in trying to distinguish onset of delirium from dementia with Lewy bodies also warrants further investigation.

While haloperidol, with its limited anticholinergic and sedative properties, has been considered the drug of choice for psychotic symptoms associated with delirium, there is a small but growing literature suggesting a role for the atypical antipsychotic agents in the management of this disorder, although to date there have been no randomized controlled trials. The possible role of cholinesterase inhibitors in the management of this challenging disorder also warrants urgent attention from the research community. The fact that delirium sits at the interface between psychiatry, neurology, and geriatric medicine should be regarded as an opportunity for collaboration rather than (as it has to date) a barrier to successful research endeavors.

In Chapter 12, Ames reminds us that most of the studies on depression with psychotic features have compared patients of all ages, usually with nonpsychotic depressed patients. Although sometimes included, elderly patients have not been the specific focus of studies in this area. And yet psychotic depression in the elderly is a severe and disabling condition with high suicide risk and a very low rate of spontaneous recovery. Also, it is a condition quite commonly seen by old age psychiatrists in clinical practice. Although the evidence base supports electroconvulsive therapy (ECT) as the most efficacious treatment for psychotic depression, physical co-morbidity precluding a general anesthetic may limit its use in the elderly. With regard to the use of pharmacotherapy for psychotic depression in the elderly, Ames demonstrates that the evidence is still limited, but that the quality of studies and their findings is improving. Most importantly, future research needs to address the problematic issue of relapse prevention in psychotic depression. Clinical guidelines are required for the doses and relative usefulness of individual antidepressants, antipsychotics, and mood-stabilizing agents, as well as for maintenance ECT.

Bipolar affective disorder (BAD) in later life imposes a substantial burden on patients, their families, and health care providers, as it can be chronic, associated with significant suicidality, and increasingly refractory to treatment. In Chapter 13 Sajatovic and Gyulai highlight the fact that important research issues which still need to be addressed include the identification of criteria for the 10% of BAD that emerges in later life, the overlap between late-onset BAD and secondary mania, and factors influencing the course and prognosis of this disabling disorder. In particular, there is a dearth of studies that have specifically examined treatment options for older patients with BAD. Despite the extensive use of lithium and sodium valproate in late-life mania, the evidence base largely has been extrapolated from mixed populations or retrospective, naturalistic studies.

The occurrence of psychotic symptoms in elderly people with dementia is a major reason for psychiatric consultation, acute hospitalization, transfer to a more intensive level of care, and prescription of powerful psychotropic medications. In Chapter 14 Douglas and Ballard outline the woeful extent of our ignorance about what works safely for the management of people in this situation. Their justifiably conservative approach to the use of medications could usefully be emulated by practitioners around the world, whose practice leads to the exposure of huge numbers of vulnerable elderly people in institutions to medications of proven toxicity and largely unproven efficacy.

The association between stressors and psychotic symptoms in the elderly has increasing clinical relevance in our aging developed societies but, to date, has received minimal research attention. In Chapter 15 Bonwick highlights the important point that, despite the widely held perception in the general community that the elderly are increasingly the victims of crime, the burgeoning literature on acute stress reactions to trauma focuses largely on younger victims. On the other hand, chronic post-traumatic stress disorder (PTSD) in the elderly is better recognized as the cohorts of veterans from the wars of the last century have aged and presented to psychiatric services with a diversity of trauma-related psychiatric sequelae. However, despite their growing numbers, research into the symptom profile (which can be very complex) of elderly patients experiencing PTSD over many decades is exceedingly limited. Further, although antipsychotic medication is commonly used to treat exacerbations of symptoms in PTSD, there has been minimal research in specific regard to elderly people with PTSD.

Whelan highlights the lack of attention to substance use and abuse in the elderly in Chapter 16. When psychosis is the consequence of alcohol abuse, it becomes obvious to clinicians. However, what are the risk factors for alcohol abuse in individual communities and are there effective prevention strategies so that the elderly will be managed well before alcohol abuse and its consequential psychotic symptoms occur? Can the primary care physician be provided with the necessary tools for preventative actions?

In Chapter 17 Chiu highlights the importance of the basal ganglia in the occurrence of psychotic symptoms in a range of disorders affecting older patients. Those who taught us that the basal ganglia were just there to control movement appear to have underestimated their multiple roles.

Having reviewed the issue of iatrogenesis in Chapter 18, Olver and Norman raise the pressing question as to how this may be reduced. Research into effective education of general practitioners and specialists has yet to be delivered.

While they are ideologically and intuitively sound, educational programs for improvement in prescribing practices have yet to be tested for long-term effectiveness.

Polypharmacy in prescribing for the elderly continues to be the rule rather than the exception in general practice and in hospital inpatient services, leading to the very unsatisfactory situation of elderly patients developing iatrogenic psychotic symptoms. On the other hand, is monotherapy of adequate efficacy to replace polypharmacy? Is there evidence that monotherapy is of superior efficacy to polypharmacy in the elderly? Even though we do see the psychoses consequent upon iatrogenesis, what are the best measures to take to prevent such sequelae?

In editing this book, the three editors have been impressed both by the extent of ignorance in regard to the etiologies of and best management strategies for psychoses affecting older people. However, we have been excited by the efforts of individual research groups and trust that the publication of this book will do something to spur further endeavors to help the clinical community better understand and manage this common and distressing array of clinical phenomena.

References

Förstl H, Burns A, Levy R et al, Neuropathological correlates of psychotic phenomena in confirmed Alzheimer's disease, *Br J Psychiatry* (1994) **165**:53–9.

Howard R, Rabins PV, Seeman MV, for the International Late-Onset Schizophrenia Group, Late onset schizophrenia and very late onset schizophrenia like psychosis: an international consensus, *Am J Psychiatry* (2000) **157**:172–8.

Index

Page numbers in *italics* indicate figures or tables